DOLLY D. GAHAGAN

SWITCH DOWN &QUIT

*What the Cigarette Companies
Don't Want You to Know
About Smoking*

SPECIAL CUT-OUT SECTION
INCLUDED

🔟 *Ten Speed Press*

1☉
TEN SPEED PRESS
P.O. Box 7123
Berkeley, California 94707

Book Design by Nancy Austin
Cover Design by Fifth Street Design Associates
Cover Illustration by Tom Weller
Typeset by Designer Type

Library of Congress Cataloging in Publication Data
Gahagan, Dolly.
  Switch down and quit.
    1. Cigarette habit—United States.   2. Cigarette
  habit—United States—Prevention.   Cigarette
  industry—United States.   I. Title.
  HV5763.G34   1987   613.8'5   86-30161
  ISBN 0-89815-204-6

Printed in the United States of America

1   2   3   4   5   —   90 98 88 87

C O N T E N T S

Purpose & Dedication

The purpose of this book is to help people who want to stop smoking.

There is an easy way to do it. The people who work for the cigarette companies and their advertising agencies told me about it. It is not entirely painless, but it is, mathematically, 99 percent easier than the cold-turkey, white-knuckle method that my husband and I were trying to use. I discovered it only because I had worked on studies for cigarette companies for over twenty years, and when my husband had his own market research firm one of his largest clients was a major manufacturer of cigarettes.

An effective method for giving up cigarettes, like the one described in this book, is one of the two things the cigarette companies really fear (the other is government legislation). The manufacturers know that psychologists and Smoke Enders cessation programs are too expensive for most people and that a very high percentage of smokers go back to smoking when their courses are done, anyway. They are also aware that most smokers are so blinded by their addiction that they rationalize away the warnings published by the Surgeon General, the American Cancer Society, the American Lung Association and the Heart Association.

The cigarette manufacturers know that if you are a smoker and you carefully follow the few simple rules given in this book, you can succeed in quitting. The key word here is **carefully.** The manufacturers are aware of the problem of losing their customers, and they are very, very savvy about keeping their business. They know about this method, they know how it works, and many of their marketing practices are designed to confuse you and make you fail. Their tricks are very effective, but you can avoid them once you know how they work. I will get into the specifics in the chapters on "How to Quit" and "Tricks and Traps."

Once you know **how** to quit, it is easy to do, as long as you follow my simple rules. There are master lists in this book that you can cut out and carry with you, so you have the basic information when you need a quick consultation.

It makes me angry as I write to think that it took us so long to quit when we knew better. My husband and I knew most of the facts, but as they say out West, we were blindsided by our addiction. We knew the data. We understood the dangers of smoking, but we kept right on smoking because we always needed "just one more cigarette." Given the amount we smoked and with our families' predisposition toward cancer, we are just plain lucky to be alive and healthy. We really knew the facts because we had done so much research for the cigarette companies' marketing departments, and we had no excuse. It would have been ironic justice if one of us had gotten lung cancer.

I want to dedicate this book to the people I love and who have helped me, such as my friend Dona at the *New York Times,* who first took the time to read this book and to offer her opinions, and my brother-in-law, Bill, who is so loyal and such a tower of strength to the whole family. Finally, I want to dedicate the book to the millions of smokers out there who want to quit and who need help; who do not know all the whys and wherefores and who struggle with their addictions without knowing what to do to relieve them.

So, smokers of America, this book is dedicated to you. I know the gut-wrenching addiction you suffer, because I used to smoke myself, and I too was humiliated by my inability to give it up.

SPECIAL NOTE

The FTC stopped publishing tar/nicotine figures in the spring of 1986. Since then, ten out of twelve of the tar/nicotine changes I could identify have been **up.** Almost every brand that changed has increased its tar/nicotine addiction level!!

Why I Know the Easy Way

*F*or the past twenty years, my husband and I have been engaged in consumer market research; at one time or another, we have participated in studies for most of the cigarette companies. Much of my work was done for advertising agencies and I also worked for my husband's survey business, Gahagan Research Associates, Inc., in New York, which specialized in consumer packaged goods research. We worked for a large variety of companies, most of them in the food and drug business, testing their products and their advertising for acceptance among consumers. Among his clients was the Brown and Williamson Tobacco Company, which makes Kool, Viceroy, Raleigh, Belair and Barclay cigarettes. In fact, after he had lost the account, my husband attempted to regain this business by creating and giving the company a detailed product development and marketing plan for a new cigarette that became the Barclay brand. Although Barclays have been almost off the market for the past several years, because of FTC problems, they were one of the most successful cigarette new product entries in twenty years. I will tell you why they are practically off the market in Chapter 5 where I discuss Tricks and Traps. Brown and Williamson changed his plan and went just a hair too far with their filters and they trapped themselves; even their usually friendly competitors were driven to cry "foul."

Cigarette sales are extremely profitable, and Brown and Williamson spent a great deal of money to research smoker attitudes. My husband's company had a total of thirty-five people working on their account alone, and this was not the company's only, or even their biggest, supplier of research. But we did do a great deal of their basic marketing research work.

Because cigarettes are so profitable, the companies can afford to, and do, research every facet of their marketing and advertising. They not only test new advertising campaigns but also minor variations in a theme. For example, they will test a menthol cigarette magazine advertisement to determine whether to use a smaller or a bigger waterfall, whether or not to include a person with the waterfall, and which of two minutely different copy versions to include. Also, since the Surgeon General's report shows that proportionately more black than white Americans smoke, every facet has to be tested among black as well as white smokers. We also tested proposed new packages and advertising campaigns for Belair and package changes for Viceroy. Since Brown and Williamson is one of the biggest users of premiums in the country, we studied how premiums can stimulate brand loyalty. The bulk of the work, however, was in new product research. We tested new names and packages for new cigarette brands, logo variations and the effects of giveaways to attract new customers. We did the test market sales research on Arctic Lights, a new menthol brand that was being test marketed in Cincinnati and Dayton. (It failed in test market.)

I have a great deal of personal respect for the marketing and research people I dealt with at Brown and Williamson and the other cigarette companies I have worked with. They are very professional and their research is extremely thorough. They study in detail every move and every possible contingency that can affect their business.

In my experience, this thoroughness goes far beyond the usual marketing tactics of testing the effects of package or advertising changes and extends to all aspects of their management planning. Nowhere is this better illustrated than in a study we did for one of the largest cigarette companies. At one point the company was concerned that the Surgeon General might be coming out with a dramatic special report on the dangers of carbon monoxide poisoning from cigarette smoke. (Carbon monoxide, as almost everyone knows, is a deadly poison.) Wanting to know in advance what the public's reaction would be to the rumored report, they asked us to design a study for them.

The key to success in any research study of this type is to make the information about the sample report appear as true to life as possible to the people you interview. We designed a study that used real copies of *Time* magazine, into which we inserted specially prepared pages with an article describing the hypothetical report. All this demanded split-second timing so that we could deliver our copies of *Time*, with the imaginary article, to respondents before the regular issues of the magazine hit the newsstands.

Two days before they reached the newsstands, we bought 1,000 hot-off-the-press issues of *Time* from the wholesalers. Our client had had special centerfold pages printed in *Time*'s format. These pages contained the imaginary article, which they had commissioned, describing the warnings in the hypothetical Surgeon General's report on the dangers of carbon monoxide. (The company was well aware of the health dangers of carbon monoxide and hired a special "safe" freelance writer to prepare the article to their specifications. We paid the writer, however. He was officially under contract to our firm in case *Time* magazine or the Surgeon General took offense at our study.) We inserted the pages into our copies of *Time* on a Sunday night and quickly gave them to smokers to read before copies of the real issue of *Time* hit the newsstands on Tuesday morning. The special pages were printed in one city, the magazines were purchased and the inserting was done in New York, and the study was conducted in Phoenix, Arizona. It was a wild night and day getting that study into the field.

The next step was to reinterview the smokers who had been given the magzines a day or two later and obtain their reactions to the article describing the warnings in the hypothetical report on carbon monoxide. Actually, it turned out that the company had been misinformed. The Surgeon General never did come out with a special report on the dangers of carbon monoxide. But since the company couldn't know that, they wanted to make sure that they would know how to protect their consumer franchise in case there was a serious negative reaction by smokers. About a year later, the Surgeon General did publish negative findings on the effects of carbon monoxide. Smokers' reactions were just as we predicted, and so the company was prepared at that time.

This study is an example of professional, forward-looking, defensive strategic planning at its best. It is the kind of protective measure that is taught at business schools but seldom ever done in real life. Most other companies would have waited until after the report came out to do their research. Our client acted before the report to protect themselves. Waiting and reacting after the fact is usually too late, because of the time it takes to do the research and to develop a strategy. It leaves management flying by the seat of its pants in a blizzard of adverse press reports, wondering what they should do next. In a situation like this, management is forced to react publicly under pressure with its critics and the media hanging on every word.

Not counting the printing, the study cost over $40,000. The company spent the money happily, just to be prepared for a possible negative reaction to their products and to learn how best to counter its effects. They are very bright marketing and management people.

As experts in consumer research, my husband and I have been involved in cigarette companies' strategic planning, as well as their marketing and product-development decision-making process. We became familiar with the facts of the marketplace and how these facts affected management actions to increase their business by keeping people addicted to cigarettes.

I also learned how to get off cigarettes—the easy way. Now I am going to tell you how.

Smokers Are Addicted to Nicotine

*O*ne definition of being physically addicted to a substance is that the person has physical symptoms when he or she stops using it. In the section under nicotine addiction the Surgeon General's Report of 1980 states, "When habitual smokers stop smoking, they may experience a wide variety of unpleasant side effects, including craving for tobacco, irritability, restlessness, dullness, sleep disturbance, gastrointestinal disturbances, anxiety and impairment of concentration, judgment and psychomotor performance.... Additional objective signs include a decrease in heart rate and blood pressure, increased rapid eye movement sleep, and slower rhythms in the EEG. Spontaneous jaw clenching lasting several weeks has been correlated with verbal reports of irritability."

The marketing and the research people at the cigarette companies are not naive. They know that they are in the fortunate position of having customers who are addicted to their product. It would be impossible if they did not know it. They love it. A brand manager said to me one day when he was particularly pleased with his job that it's a great business, really. What other job could he have where his customers were so addicted to his products that they couldn't work, sleep, write, run a house, do almost anything without their daily "fix."

5

This attitude was also clear in a conversation about a new menthol cigarette one of my clients was introducing. The black market is extremely important to this company. Blacks are responsible for over 50 percent of menthol cigarette sales, and their flagship brand is a menthol cigarette. It supports the company. Without this brand and its black market sales, the company would have problems maintaining its share of market. However, they did not have a lock on the black market. Salem, the menthol market entry put out by the giant R.J. Reynolds Tobacco Company, was closing in and gradually reducing their leadership among blacks. This was of major concern to the company because Reynolds is five times the size of my client and could throw virtually unlimited dollars against them in an effort to buy customers.

The client wanted to do something to stop the erosion of its market or else gain new menthol customers from other areas. They decided to develop a new brand that would compete directly against Salem in its home territory—white male menthol cigarette smokers. This brand was to be aimed right straight at the average midwestern white American and it was to be test marketed in Dayton and Cincinnati, Ohio. We were chosen to do the market research survey that tracked its sales and the penetration of its advertising and promotion campaigns in the two introductory test markets. It was a big job involving over 80,000 phone calls.

There was a very aggressive, blunt, hard-driving young woman involved with the new product introductory program. She stated the fact of addiction in a terse, dramatic way as she tried to describe the kind of smokers that were her target market group for the introductory campaign. She just boldly said, "We've got 'em hooked."

Another corporate executive spoke plainly about addiction, and brought it home to me as we were sitting around his swimming pool in the suburbs. He pointed out that his company never tries to sell people on smoking, because they don't need to. Taking that approach would only draw fire from lots of the anti-smoking groups. People are addicted to cigarettes. "Like you," he said to my husband. "You're an addict."

But, he cautioned us, we were never to mention the word "addict" around the company, and if we did, we would risk losing them as a client. They wanted to be sure no politicians got the material to hang a tag on them as selling an addictive product.

But it is no secret to most smokers that they are addicted to cigarettes. When they try to stop, they go crazy with withdrawal symptoms. Suddenly the only thing that they can think about is a cigarette, or a pipe, or a cigar, or Bantron, the nicotine chewing gum or anything that will get this awful monkey of desire off their backs. One brand manager who smokes consoled my husband about his unsuccessful efforts to give up smoking by reminding him he was just like everyone else caught up in that physical yearning. They're tough to give up, he said; believe me, you will walk a mile for a Camel, or any other cigarette you happen to like. You will walk two miles, or maybe five miles, and you will come back with a carton because you don't want to be without your fix again. You may not run, but as the store comes within view, you will walk a lot faster because you absolutely have to satisfy that addiction.

And from what I know he is right. It is a physical addiction. Now, I have all kinds of psychologist confreres in the research business who will tell you that it is not physically addictive, but only a psychological addiction. However, there was never any evidence in the research we did for tobacco companies, or in the interviews I did for this book, that indicated that the tobacco addiction was psychological. Respondents always describe it in physical terms. And the research people we have talked with at different cigarette companies have always called it a physical addiction. They laugh at the psychologists who say it is mental or psychological. I don't know of any smoker who believes it either.

This is not only my opinion. None of the research data I have ever seen nor the interviews I conducted for this book appear to bear out the hypothesis that smoking addiction is caused by psychological factors. Respondents who have tried to give up smoking almost invariably describe cigarette withdrawal pangs as a physical sensation, and often they speak of a gut-wrenching yearning that prevents them from working or getting on with their lives until it is satisfied. One respondent put it this way:

> When I tried to give up cigarettes, I was climbing the walls, I couldn't work. I couldn't concentrate or even sit still at my desk. So I went to my boss and asked him to forget about me for a week. I was giving up cigarettes and I wouldn't be good for anything. He was a nice guy and fortunately, he was an ex-smoker himself, so he went along. Thank God it was a doldrums period and there was only a very light work load. He covered for me, and did my work as well as his own, while I sat in my office and banged my head on the walls. That's a nice boss.

A New York taxi driver describes what he went through trying to get off cigarettes and still keep on the job driving a cab.

It was the hardest thing I ever tried to do. I couldn't do it again. It was like I was on drugs, or something. You swear at everybody. You yell and scream and curse. The worst part was the first two weeks. I got two tickets and I had a small accident. I never get tickets. I never bump into somebody. I even shut all the windows and screamed one day.

But even after that, every couple days I would get hit with the worst kind of awful aching for a cigarette.

I had to keep tellin' myself—'No, you will not stop the car. You will pass the store. No, you will not go in the store and buy a pack of cigarettes.' It was the most awful physical urge—and then it would pass—until the next time.

My wife said she couldn't stand it. She told me to go back to smokin'—but I wouldn't do it. I couldn't never go through that again. I would not ever touch another cigarette.

A woman explained how it affects her if she is without a cigarette even for a few hours in the morning.

The cigarette I want most is the first one in the morning. I need it or else I am just no good. I can't do anything until I have my cigarette. I don't want a cup of coffee; I don't want to talk with anyone. When the cigarettes run out I get all jumpy and nervous; and fiesty, like I'm angry. You don't want to be around me when I'm like that.

The last time it happened I ran to the store and was at work a half an hour early because the store is right by the train station. Another time, I got the urge to quit and it lasted bout six minutes. I need that lift in the morning.

A senior vice-president of a brokerage house said:

It was a very difficult thing for me to do. I smoke all day at my desk. When I tried to give them up, I think I would have smoked anything. I almost started smoking a pipe, but I decided that wouldn't do any good. I would still be hooked. A client offered me a cigar one day at lunch at the Harvard Club. I wanted that cigar so badly, my hand was shaking. Did I smoke it? No, it's still in my desk. I keep it there to remind myself never to smoke.

An executive secretary described how disgusted she was when she discovered how hung up she was on cigarettes.

We had to work late one night on a big report. We ran out and the stores were closed. You want to know something: I went around the whole office smoking butts out of ashtrays. That's disgusting. That's how bad I am. I'm hooked; and the worst part about it is, I know it and I can't quit. I try to cut down, but I get so nervous I can't do the typing or the petty cash, or if I am at a party, I need it then; it's worse in the morning, if there's not one there I snap at my guy. I need 'em and I just can't cut it out.

It just won't let me drop the habit.

A friend of ours reminded me of what an alcoholic once told me. He said something like, "Smoking is an addiction just like drinking. There's always an excuse to drink. An alcoholic will drink if he's happy, he will drink if he's sad; we will drink to celebrate, we will drink if we fail; we will drink because it's a party and we will drink because we are alone. For us, there is always a reason to drink."

And for us, there was always a reason to smoke. My excuse for smoking was that I needed a cigarette when I was with people. My husband's excuse was that he needed cigarettes to cope with a nasty, demanding client who enjoyed making his life miserable at work (sometimes it seemed like twenty-four hours a day). He thought that reaching for a cigarette gave him time to think. Actually it was just a rationalization, an excuse to make his smoking permissible so that he would not have to face the frustration of stopping. It was our own way of kidding ourselves about our cigarette addiction.

A middle-management executive in the Midwest said that when she tried to stop smoking, just the smell of the smoke from someone else's cigarette could be irresistible.

My husband and I both used cigarettes. I tried to give them up but I couldn't. We would be watching television, and I would be trying not to think about how much I wanted a cigarette and then he would light one. I would smell the smoke and it would trigger a craving for a cigarette. I mean a real physical craving. It was too much to resist. Anyway, it was too much for me to resist. It is terribly frustrating because you ought to be able to stop. As soon as you smell the smoke, it is just like a magnet. It grabs you and pulls you and you have no control over yourself.

Another respondent told me how he continues to smoke, although his wife will not let him smoke in the house and makes him go out in the cold.

The trouble is, that now I have an awful problem in quitting. My wife doesn't smoke. She hates smoking. She says it makes the whole house smell. Sometimes she makes me go out of the house to smoke, even in winter. I feel guilty about it because I know it is bad for me but I have tried to quit 50 times and I can't do it. The urge is too great. I can't stop. Yes, I have to go outside in the winter if I want to smoke. She makes me feel like a bad child but I do it anyway because I want that cigarette so bad.

The owner of a large industrial trucking company described how he tried everything, even a hypnotist, to get off smoking.

I am ashamed to admit this but I can't get off smoking. I started years ago, when I was a kid in Chicago. I know that it isn't good for me. I'm no fool. I own a big business. My wife is always after me to quit. But I couldn't do it. I finally went to a hypnotist. I went to him three times before he hypnotized me. He said I was very difficult. Well, he hypnotized me three times, and I gave them up for six weeks. Why did I go back? We had a strike—the Teamsters. We were losing money like, terrible. I had one. Before I knew it I had smoked the pack and then I was hooked again. I was mad, but I'm not going back to that hypnotist. I don't trust those people. Who knows what they might ask you when they got you like that?

A blue-collar respondent summed it up this way:

There ain't nothing psychological about it. You gotta have one because you can't stop. How do I feel? I get itchy. I feel nervous and bothered. My muscles don't work right. I just gotta have a smoke.

There are many nicotine substitutes that people use to try to get off cigarettes. For example, there is Bantron, a nicotine chewing gum available on prescription. But as anyone who has used it knows, it doesn't work. The nicotine in a nicotine chewing gum will stop the pangs of desire for a cigarette, but that doesn't solve the problem. You are still addicted to nicotine. It is just that instead of having the satisfaction of nicotine in a cigarette, the chewer has the satisfaction of nicotine in a piece of gum. The user is still hooked.

Many smokers do not see themselves as addicts, much less drug addicts. This is both a cultural and an ego problem. In our society it is not socially permissible to be an addict, because the word "addict" implies that the person takes illegal narcotic or psychoactive drugs, things like cocaine, heroin, LSD, or angel dust.

Most people do not call an alcoholic an addict, even though the alcoholic is certainly addicted to alcohol, often with devastating personal effects. The words "addict" and "addicted" connote the illegal drug culture and not legally sold, addictive products such as cigarettes and alcohol.

Let's face it, certain people probably are mildly addicted to chocolate.

Among our respondents, just the connotation of being addicted to cigarettes raised the hackles on some smokers.

I am not an addict. I wouldn't give you ten cents for every drug addict in New York. You can go to Hell.

I can give up cigarettes any time I want to. I tried to quit but I like them, but I am not an addict.

Another respondent said:

Where I am, an addict is someone who is on drugs. He's addicted. He's gotta have his fix. They'll do anything for it. They'll kill you (for a fix). That's how bad it is.

A blue-collar respondent said:

I ain't no addict. Addicts is criminals. I like to smoke. There's nothin' wrong with that.

One woman summed it up like this:

I guess I am addicted to cigarettes if you mean I'm in the habit of smoking and I can't seem to give them up. But I don't think of myself as a drug addict. I don't think anyone who smokes thinks of themselves that way.

In a large sense, the word addiction is so closely associated with hard drugs that the negative connotations are understandable. On a deeper level, I suspect that society sees nothing wrong with a product such as cigarettes being addictive, as long as it does not drive people to crime in order to satisfy their addiction. That is society's attitude toward alcohol. The addictive nature of cigarettes will never rouse the concern of the public as long as it **only** affects the smoker. So it is up to the individual to determine the consequences of his addiction—and they are severe, as the chapter on the dangers of smoking makes clear. And only you, the smoker, can decide to act on your own behalf and kick the nicotine habit.

Despite all smokers' rationalizations to the contrary, smoking is an addiction. When you stop smoking, you experience some very uncomfortable physical effects. Thanks to what we learned about the management of nicotine addiction from the professionals who want to keep you addicted, we figured out how to get off tobacco the easy way, to minimize the pangs of withdrawal and make it possible for us to improve our odds of a long and healthy life. Yes, you are addicted. Yes, you can stop. Get to know your addiction, and you can take the first step to ending it.

In the next chapter I describe how addiction works, and then I lay out the simple method you can use to quit smoking.

How Your Addiction Works

There are many systems for giving up cigarettes. For us, none of them worked. We had to figure out a method that did. Anyone who has worked for cigarette companies or on cigarette studies at advertising agencies as long as we have (twenty-six years) knows that quackery in abundance is thrown around about quitting cigarettes, probably more than about anything else except dieting.

One of the big problems with most methods of quitting smoking is recidivism. They hold your hand while you are trying to give cigarettes up, but then when you do quit, they let go and you dive back in and start smoking all over again. They do not teach you how to stay off, because you don't know why or how badly you are hooked.

We are going to teach you that. But facts alone are not enough. To get a smoker off cigarettes, you have to be able to translate facts into actions that a person can use in his or her daily life. That is the nitty gritty, the bottom line or whatever you want to call it. My own personal question is, "Does it work in the real world, when it is out there all alone and trying to survive in the cold?" My method works, but you will have to be careful and go slowly.

LEVEL OF ADDICTION

The first practical step to take is to figure out your level of addiction. From there on, switching down is a simple, logical, step-by-step action that you will take every three weeks. One step follows along after another. That is what makes our method so easy. The main question for the smoker trying to get off cigarettes is: "How badly am I hooked?"

A couple of examples will show you what I mean by level of addiction. Since the most popular brand in the country is Marlboro, I will start with this brand because people are most familiar with it.

It is very important to be precise, and so I will specify that our Marlboro user smokes one package a day of King Size (that is, 85 millimeters long) Marlboros in the soft package.

Why am I being so precise about the kind of package, the length and all of that? You must get used to it. This is how I am going to get you off cigarettes the easy way. If you are a smoker, you are addicted to a certain amount of nicotine. But you must remember that the amount of nicotine varies by the **type, the length and even the package** of the cigarette brand you smoke.

All right, our Marlboro smoker smokes one pack of King Size (85-millimeter) Marlboros in the soft pack per day. That is 20 cigarettes. Each Marlboro has 1.0 milligrams of nicotine. That means his addiction level is 20.0 milligrams of nicotine per day (20 × 1.0).

If he were smoking King Size (85-millimeter) Merits in a soft pack, his addiction level would be 10.0. Merits are a milder cigarette, with a nicotine level of only .5 milligrams per cigarette; .5 times 20 cigarettes equals 10.0 milligrams of nicotine per day. So this smoker is addicted at about half the level of the Marlboro smoker.

Now, let us take a smoker who smokes Now cigarettes. According to the Surgeon General's report, the nicotine level of a Now, soft-pack, 85-millimeter cigarette is .1. That number, .1, times 20 cigarettes per day means that this smoker has an addiction level of 2.0 milligrams of nicotine per day.

All right, let us review what we have just read. We have three smokers, each of whom smokes the 85-millimeter soft-package version of a brand. They have different levels of addiction to nicotine.

These are the facts. The "pack-a-day" smoker is addicted to that many milligrams of nicotine depending on the brand, just as the

ADDICTION LEVELS

(1 pack a day)

Brand	Nicotine per Cigarette	Addiction Level
Marlboro King Size, Soft Pack	1.0	20.0
Merit King Size, Soft Pack	.5	10.0
Now King Size, Soft Pack	.1	2.0

crack user is addicted to his or her quota of cocaine. Fortunately, with our method it is easier for the smoker to get off cigarettes than it is for a crack user to get off cocaine—even though you may not think so right now.

All right. You tell me, if each of these three smokers were to give up smoking, who would have the easier time of it.

You guessed it. The Now smoker.

Next, tell me which of these three smokers would have the hardest time. Right. The Marlboro smoker.

What the Cigarette Companies Know About Dropping Nicotine Levels

Great, you say to yourself, all I have to do is to drop my level of nicotine intake a couple of times and I can quit.

Not that easy. Unless you know how much to drop, how often to drop and what to drop to, the chances are you will not make it. You may even bounce back up where you were.

The funny thing is that the cigarette companies were faced with much the same problem, but for a different reason. What they did and what they found out can be a very big help to you in giving up cigarettes.

With all of the uproar in the media and government about the health hazards of smoking, it inevitably occurred to smokers that it would be healthier for them if they were to smoke a lower tar/nicotine level cigarette. The cigarette companies realized that if they did not want to lose these "health concerned" smokers, they would have to produce an alternate that their customers could smoke. Thus, the birth of "Light" cigarettes: Marlboro Lights, Kool Lights, Winston Lights, Kent Golden Lights, etc.

However, before they took this step, a company had to do some basic research. They needed to know how much they could reduce the nicotine level of a brand without having a customer feel frustrated enough to switch to another brand. This is a very important question to a cigarette company, and they were not aobut to try to solve it in a hit-or-miss fashion. If they were to reduce the nicotine level of a brand too much, they could lose a lot of their customers— for two reasons. First of all, changing the nicotine level could affect customer satisfaction. Smokers, perhaps not even noticing the change in nicotine level, could feel frustrated by the new cigarette, possibly become dissatisfied, and then switch brands. Second, changing the nicotine levels would also mean changing the tar levels, and that invariably would change the taste; this change also might cause dissatisfaction serious enough to result in brand switching, and any loss in regular customers is very serious in the cigarette business.

Believe it or not, the difficulty the cigarette companies faced was that smokers do not switch around very much from one brand to another. Because of the image identification factor, most customers are extremely loyal to their cigarette brands and very seldom change the basic brand they buy. (The main switching is to and from a menthol brand alternate with similar image connotations.) However, this extreme brand loyalty is a two-edged sword. It also means that if you ever lose a customer, it is very expensive (perhaps up to $300 per customer) to get him or her back. Once the customer has left your brand and gone to another, the brand loyalty factor works against you instead of for you.

The enormous expense of getting a customer is one of the main reasons why changing anything about a product or marketing program is always such a traumatic affair for management. It is also the reason that management in the tobacco business is so consumer-research conscious and that every little change in a product, a package or an advertisement is pretested. The purpose is not only to see if a change will attract new customers, but also to make sure that it does not alienate any of its present loyal customer base.

Since a cigarette company works tremendously hard to build a loyal core of customers, it is not hard to understand their fears, given the recent example of what happened to Coca-Cola. Coca-Cola changed their formula, and they very nearly lost most of their customers. They had to scramble back to market with the old version, now called "Coke Classic," and attempt to recapture their customers. Coke is a very strong brand, and management was able to move quickly enough so that they didn't lose too many customers. However, it was a nightmarish situation for the company. It is conceivable that a wrong product change, such as the one Coca-Cola masterminded, could have put a weaker brand out of business. However, that is not likely to happen at the cigarette companies because their consumer research managements are much too sophisticated to allow it. (Coca-Cola has always had a very weak market research department.)

What the cigarette companies did in order to solve their problem was to order a large amount of blind product testing. Blind product testing involved giving smokers different cigarettes marked only with a letter, such as "L" or "R," and having them smoke them for a period of time, usually a week or two. Then they re-interview the smokers using a telephone call-back after a few days to give the respondent time to use and compare the test product to his usual brand under real-life circumstances. This gives the research people a chance to find out smokers' preferences, their reasons for preference and other information describing their likes and dislikes for a test formula. The companies are very conscious of their product quality and this type of research is usually the largest single item in their whole consumer-research budget.

Going ahead with the blind product testing meant that the cigarette brand managers, who live and die by their brand's share of market, watching their sales figures daily with almost microscopic care, would know in advance what smokers' reactions would be to a drop in the tar/nicotine levels.

At any rate, here is what I was told they discovered by people who worked for research suppliers of two of the big tobacco companies.

They could reduce the nicotine levels of a cigarette by about 2 to 3 milligrams or 20 percent, whichever is less, without smokers being aware of the reduction.

Isn't that a wonderful piece of information? That single finding, in a few words, tells you how to develop a plan for quitting without discomfort, or at least with only minor discomfort.

For the poor, sitting-duck smoker who really wants to quit, it is a perfectly marvelous research finding.

I would like to say I had worked on these studies, but let me hasten to say that we didn't do the work. They were done by another supplier and we heard about the results one day at lunch. Our company was growing, and we needed some additional people, so we were trying to hire an old friend for our staff. Without being the least bit aware of it, we were, in fact, trying to hire the agency research liaison man who had been assigned to the tar/nicotine reduction studies for a competitive company.

Because it held out the possibility of more work for us, we naturally told our tobacco client what we had learned. They said that they had already done the same kinds of studies, although they were pleased to learn what we were telling them paralleled the findings of their product-testing supplier.

People Aren't Stupid But They Can Be Confused

The whole episode reinforced a conviction I have had for many years. I believe that no one is smarter about products and what they want out of them than the people who use them. In saying this, I am not talking about individuals, because individuals really may not be that smart. I am talking about the public as a whole. In the mass, it is impossible to sell the public something it does not want on a continuing basis. You may be able to do it once, but you can never do it twice, and no manufacturer can stay in business on a "one-time sale." People just will not take their money out of their pockets to pay for something that they do not want. It is that simple.

Now, because people aren't dumb, they could plainly see that they could switch brands and lessen their addiction. The cigarette companies knew it too. They told us that customer loss through switching down was the one thing that they really feared from their customers. Unless something could be done to stop smokers from switching brands and steadily dropping their tar/nicotine levels, so many customers would switch down, and then out, that it could well put a severe crimp in the cigarette business. From the cigarette companies' point of view, the really terrible thing was that some people were already reducing their addiction levels to the point where it made it easy for them to quit smoking.

That may sound strange to you, to call this a terrible trend, but when you are a brand marketing manager and your livelihood depends on how many cigarettes you can sell, the thought of people quitting smoking is pretty horrendous. The companies had to do something to stop the trend and prevent smokers from switching down and out. It had to be done legally and quickly, and they couldn't let smokers know about it.

And they did all of these things: They carried on careful market research. The anticipated consumer reactions. And they developed techniques they could use to confuse smokers about the tar/nicotine levels of the brands and types they were smoking. And it worked. It has dramatically slowed the drain of people quitting.

So, don't think you know how to quit—because you don't, **yet.** You may have a general idea of what to do, but that is it. Since the cigarette companies have done so much research, they know just how to confuse you and to trap you into smoking at a nicotine level high enough to keep you addicted. They have already:

- Done the consumer research to determine how to trap you.

- Pretested the traps that will trick you into smoking a strong enough version of a brand to keep you addicted.

- Market tested the methods to make sure they work in fact as well as in theory. (They work like a charm.)

- Put the whole plan into operation nationally.

The problem is that unless you know the tricks they use to keep you addicted, you can inadvertently smoke such a strong cigarette that it will be too hard for you to quit. I will go into details later, but for right now, just let me give you two hints.

In one Ultra Low Tar brand, one size cigarette is **6 times as strong** as another size, and a cigarette in one kind of package is **10 times as strong** as the same size cigarette in another kind of package.

These are only two of the ways they bounce you back up to a higher nicotine intake just when you have your addiction down low enough to get off cigarettes without driving yourself up a wall. This is why I say that you will have to go slowly and pay careful attention to my warnings, if you want to quit cigarettes the easy way.

By now, you should understand that if you smoke, you are

addicted to nicotine at a certain level. The higher the nicotine content of the cigarette you smoke, the stronger your addiction and the longer it will take (but it will not be any harder) to break yourself of your habit.

That is the nitty gritty. You have to face the fact that you are an addict.

How to Quit

*N*ow, since the purpose of this book is to get you off smoking the easy way, let us use the information we have to start you on the road to quitting the easy way.

We all know the hard way. The anger, frustration, the irritation, the desire that drives us out of the house, into the car and to the store; that will not let us work or play or rest or sleep; that makes our body's hunger for a cigarette fill up our mind until it seems as though our very soul is possessed; the relief that comes as we drown ourselves in the sweet satisfaction that comes with the first puff of smoke as it swirls softly into every corner of our lungs.

Well, you are not going to have to go through any of that. You are going to smoke and enjoy it until you quit—and even then it won't be too bad.

My method calls for you to gradually reduce the amount of tar/nicotine to which you are addicted. The key word here is **gradually,** because the faster that you try to quit smoking, the more likely you are to become frustrated and therefore fail. In short, we are going to show you how to gradually wean yourself of the habit. You will do it slowly. If you follow the rules, you won't notice anything more than minor taste dissatisfaction. You will smoke a bit more each time you slowly cut down on your nicotine intake, but the market researchers have learned that you will have a minimum of discomfort. Meanwhile your total nicotine intake will gradually diminish and your level of addiction will recede to the point where you can smoke or not smoke, as you desire.

It sounds easy. It is easy.

Just be sure to follow the rules, but most of all, when you ask for your brand and type of cigarette at the store ... do it CAREFULLY ... very CAREFULLY. You must ask for exactly the brand and SIZE and PACKAGE I specify, and you MUST NOT take substitutes.

I have laid out a plan for you to follow, no matter what brand and type of cigarettes you smoke right now. The design of the plan is based on a number of factors. First, there is the principle that if you drop at the rate of only 2 to 3 milligrams of tar or .2 to .3 milligrams of nicotine at a time, you will have a maximum of smoking enjoyment and a minimum of discomfort.

The second factor the plan considers is taste. Why is taste important in selecting what brand, type and package to switch to next? Well, it will take a minute to tell you, but it is something you should know if you want to quit. The reason is that, by and large, tobacco companies specialize in one of two different approaches to creating a good tobacco taste. It all started many years ago and is rooted in the history of the tobacco business. At one time there were two major tobacco companies, the American Tobacco Company and The R.J. Reynolds Tobacco Company. The American Tobacco Company treated and also flavored its tobacco to improve its taste. Since Mr. George Washington Hill, their chairman of the board at the time, was a famous advertising genius, they used their special treatment of tobacco as a selling point to promote their brands in their advertising.

If you are old enough, you may remember the American Tobacco Company's Lucky Strike campaign, "It's Toasted." It was the centerpiece of their advertising in the days prior to World War II, and it made Lucky Strike one of the largest-selling brands of cigarettes in the United States at that time. On the other hand, R.J. Reynolds created a different taste formulation for its brands that relied more heavily upon the natural flavor of stronger-tasting tobaccos, such as Burley, for the flavor in its brands. Thus, in attempting to differentiate their brands, the two titans of the early days developed basically different taste formulations.

Now, if you were a smaller tobacco company at that time, and attempting to survive or even to grow a little without being crushed, the best that you could do was to try to nibble away at the market share of one or the other of the giants. Practical cost considerations made it impossible for you to copy both flavor formulas and it was simply too risky to go out and try to create a whole new taste configuration of your own and hope that it would appeal to smokers. So the smaller tobacco companies imitated the larger ones and specialized either in a flavored taste or a blended tobacco taste to entice consumers to their brands.

These two basic flavor approaches exist today. The giants of yesterday are not necessarily the same titans who dominate the cigarette market now, but the pattern they set still structures the taste configurations of the market. If my memory serves me correctly, Brown and Williamson and Lorillard still generally follow the R.J. Reynolds pattern of little or no flavorings. I was told in Winston-Salem that Brown and Williamson still goes to the extreme of using natural menthol, which they import all the way from Brazil, even though all their taste testing shows that menthol smokers cannot tell the difference between natural and artificial menthol flavors in the smoke. On the other hand, they told me that Phillip Morris, today's giant in the industry, follows the American Tobacco pattern of a greater use of artificial flavorings.

What is the point of all of this? Well, since you will probably be more comfortable sticking with the kind of taste you are accustomed to, I have tried to do the brand switching without jumping you back and forth from one taste configuration to the other. That way it is less likely that you will become dissatisfied with what you are smoking.

As in all things, there is an exception to this pattern. When you get down to what the manufacturers call the "Ultra Low" segment of the market, that is, cigarettes that are less than 6 milligrams of tar, two things happen. First of all, in order to reduce the amount of nicotine to less than 6 milligrams per cigarette, the manufacturers use reconstituted tobacco. This enables them to produce a leaf with much lower nicotine content. To do this, they use all of the refuse from cigarette manufacturing. They grind up all the stems, tobacco dust and leaf tendons from their factories into a paste and then roll it out into new leaves. By making the reconstituted tobacco themselves instead of buying new leaf from the farmers, they save a lot of money. Also, since the stems and the woody fibers have less nicotine content, this helps them lower the amount of nicotine in their cigarettes, while still maintaining some tobacco taste.

I have also been told that they use waste products from food-manufacturing operations. Examples of these are such things as coconut fiber, vegetable products (lettuce leaves) and cocoa fibers. The companies use these to dilute the amount of tobacco and bring the tar/nicotine levels down to the point where they will have an advertising claim. Of course, all of these ingredients are taste enhancers or adulterants depending on how you look at them. I am not condemning the cigarette companies for this. Lettuce leaves and coconut fiber are probably healthier to smoke than tobacco leaves.

In addition, when a manufacturer tries to produce an Ultra Low Tar cigarette, they are faced with a very simple fact of life. The woody fibers in reconstituted tobacco produce less "tar" when they burn. Tar creates the taste. Therefore, a less tarry smoke means a cigarette with less taste and flavor, because, without that tar, your cigarette is going to taste thin. Under these circumstances, the manufacturer has no alternative except to add flavorings if he wants to produce a viable product. At the very low tar levels, using flavorings is really the only way that the company can produce a cigarette with any taste at all. So, at a certain point, all manufacturers use flavorings.

At this point, I hasten to say that the use of flavorings has always been widespread in the tobacco business. Menthol and various mint/menthol flavors are, of course, well known. However, most people do not know that pipe tobacco and plug chewing tobacco are now and have always been about one-third sugar. Some brands also have more or less of a molasses flavor depending upon the grade of sugar and the amount of molasses used by the manufacturer. In addition to pipe and plug tobacco, many cigarette brands also have some sugar, although much less than pipe and plug tobacco. I have also heard that one of the most prevalent of the flavors is cocoa (chocolate) and that many others are used.

That is a long explanation for a simple idea, but I believe you ought to know as much as you can of the facts behind the plan I have developed for you. At least that way you won't think I am just making arbitrary decisions when I suggest a brand with a lower tar/nicotine level for you to switch to.

Now, you may well laugh at the third thing I have taken into account. But believe you me, it is very important. This factor is Brand Image. Go ahead and laugh—but while you laugh, think of this. The man who smokes non-filtered English Ovals, a very strong

American copy of an imported English cigarette, will not feel comfortable switching to Bull Durham, or Half and Half, even though they are considerably milder. Similarly, a lady who smokes Virginia Slims is probably not going to want to switch to Camel Lights, even though Camel Lights is a milder cigarette. So I have tried to pick brands that are consistent with the image of what a smoker may be smoking now.

In case my suggestions don't appeal to you, there is a do-it-yourself section later in the book, Chapter 6, from which you can make your own choices. I think that way is harder and you are more likely to run into problems, but you may find it much easier and more satisfying to make your own choices. No matter which path you elect to take, I have tried to include all the guidance you will need to quit successfuly.

SWITCHING DOWN

I am going to give you a list of 239 brands and types of cigarettes, divided into regular and menthol cigarettes. You will probably smoke one of these. First you must look up the brand and type of cigarette you are smoking in the LEFT-HAND column of the list. Opposite this, in the RIGHT-HAND column of the list, will be the name of another brand and type of cigarette for you to switch to.

You will switch your brand and type of cigarette EVERY THREE WEEKS.

At the end of three weeks, you will look up the name of the new brand you are now smoking in the LEFT-HAND column. Opposite this brand name will again be the name of another brand in the RIGHT-HAND column you should switch to. You will smoke that brand for three weeks and then switch brands again. Each time you do this, you will be lowering your tar/nicotine intake.

As soon as you switch, you will start to smoke somewhat more than your usual number of cigarettes, but this will soon level off and your smoking habits will return to your normal level of consumption. What happens in the beginning of each switch down is that your body tries to compensate for the lack of the nicotine it is getting by having you smoke more cigarettes each day. But it slowly gets used to the new level and, as it does, your need for nicotine is reduced and you return to your normal amount of smoking.

This takes about three weeks. If you try to do it in less time, it may not work, particularly if you are strongly addicted, as I was. The reason it may not work is that if you are not completely ready, your **next** drop will be very unsatisfactory. Do not forget, I have you on a constantly decreasing schedule. If you try to do it too quickly, it will become increasingly unsatisfying. If you do not follow the directions, you may end up smoking more and enjoying it less, which is something I do not want to happen. Of course, to a certain degree, you are going to be doing that anyway, but it should not be noticeable, at least not until you get down to the .4 milligrams nicotine level.

In short, if you either try to drop your tar/nicotine levels without allowing enough time for your body to become acclimated, or if you try to drop by too many milligrams at a time, you will have a slow but steady build-up of frustration. This is what I want you to avoid and you can avoid it by going in a steady methodical manner.

Take my word for it. The highest failure rates in switching down are with people who either drop too much at a time or who do not leave enough time for their addiction levels to settle down before going on to the next step. The ultimate extreme, of course, is to quit "cold turkey" the way we used to quit. But the cold-turkey treatment is pretty painful and it does not work very well. I have talked with a lot of other research people about this and we have agreed that it is because the more you increase frustration, the more you also increase desire. That leads to a lot of people going back to smoking who otherwise might not have done so. After a while, the demands of their bodies just get to them.

I have tried to depict what will happen to the number of cigarettes you smoke in a day each time you switch down in the accompanying graph. Note that your consumption will first increase as your body tries to compensate for the lack of nicotine and then level off as you gradually become satisfied with your new brand of cigarette.

It appears that a smoker returns to his previous smoking level after about fourteen days. Since that is the **average,** we expect that 50 percent of people will take longer to become adjusted and 50 percent of people will be adjusted sooner. That is one of the reasons that the plan allows more time than the average person requires. I

AUTHOR'S DIAGRAM ILLUSTRATING
CHANGE IN SMOKING CONSUMPTIONS

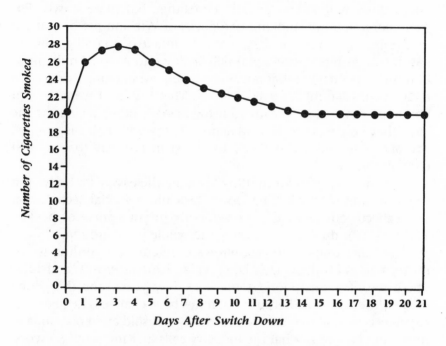

Days After Switch Down

don't want to frustrate those people who are more addicted than average. The second reason is that I cannot always create the same drop in tar/nicotine levels for you every time. Often there is no ideal option available for you to switch to; also, there are sometimes major taste and flavoring differences between manufacturers that you have to get accustomed to. Finally, there may be an ideal brand to switch to, but its sales may be so low that its distribution is poor and it is hard to find on store shelves. So, at some point, I may be picking a brand and type of cigarette for you that is less than ideal.

I am trying to make things easier for you and not more difficult; sometimes that will require a little more time with a brand on your part than average.

All right, you say, I understand all of that, but I am different. The number of cigarettes I smoked stayed high and didn't revert all the way down to the number of cigarettes I used to smoke each day. That probably won't happen, but if it does, don't worry. You will benefit the next time you drop—not necessarily the first time. The main thing is that your tar/nicotine consumption per cigarette **is** dropping, and as it continues to drop, your addiction level will drop as well.

In other words, you are still benefiting, but more slowly. For example, if you are smoking two packs of Winston per day, at 1.0 milligrams of nicotine per day, that is an intake of 40 milligrams per day. If you drop two levels, you will be down to 20 to 24 milligrams of nicotine per day. At that rate, even if you are smoking three packs a day, your total intake will be lower. That is what I want. I want you to go down slowly, with your own body's needs regulating the pace that you reduce your addiction. Everyone's habit is unique. My plan will allow your body to adjust in the way that is most comfortable for you.

Here are the rules for quitting smoking the easy way. I have put the rules and the Switching Down List into a special section that you can cut out and carry conveniently in your purse or pocket. This way, you don't have to carry the whole book around.

One final thing. The cigarettes are described according to industry names for their sizes, i.e., regular, King Size, 100s and 120s. These are old descriptions going back fifty years, and they don't make sense any more because cigarettes have changed. Regular-size cigarettes, 80 millimeters, are practically not sold anymore. Today's most popular size is what the industry calls a "King Size." So when you ask for a King Size, you are getting today's most popular, or "regular," size. Your supermarket clerk may not know them that way, but your stationer, cigar store operator and druggist will, because that is the way they order them.

THE NINE PRETESTED RULES FOR SUCCESS

1. Please follow the rules. They have been designed to help you succeed.

2. Mark your brand and type of cigarette in the left-hand column. Switch to the brand in the right-hand column. Keep doing this until you quit.

3. Be sure to buy the exact brand, size and kind of package I tell you to buy. I cannot emphasize this too much. Constantly changing the strength of cigarettes in different packages and sizes is the chief way manufacturers fool you into smoking a stronger cigarette, thereby keeping you addicted.

4. Never, never, never trade up to a higher nicotine content cigarette.

5. If your store does not carry the brand you want, have them order one or two cartons for you.

6. Do not accept an excuse like "They do not make that cigarette brand anymore." It is just because the store-keeper is too lazy to get you what you want.

7. If you must smoke a stronger cigarette because there are no others, punch holes with a pencil between the filter and the tobacco to let in more air and make the cigarette milder. Don't be embarrassed to do this if you need to.

8. Remember to switch every three weeks.

9. Always buy by the carton so you do not run out and are tempted to switch to another brand or type if your own are not available.

MASTER LIST

For Switching Down to a Lower Tar/Nicotine Level

REGULAR CIGARETTES

HOW TO USE THE LIST

1. Find your brand and type in the left-hand column. Switch down to the brand in the right-hand column.
2. Switch to a new brand every three weeks.
3. Work your way down and off the list.
   Very important! Do not substitute sizes or packages. Box and Soft Pack are almost always different strengths. King Size, 100s and 120s are almost always different strengths. If you can't find what you want, refer to the Do-It-Yourself chapter.

All brands are filter cigarettes unless marked "NF," Non-Filter.
All packages are Soft Packs unless marked "Box."

BRAND AND TYPE YOU SMOKE NOW	BRAND AND TYPE TO SWITCH TO
BARCLAY KING SIZE	NOW KING SIZE
BARCLAY KING SIZE; BOX	NOW KING SIZE
BARCLAY 100S	NOW 100S
BENSON & HEDGES; KING SIZE BOX	TAREYTON KING SIZE
BENSON & HEDGES 100S	PARLIAMENT LIGHTS 100S
BENSON & HEDGES 100S BOX	PARLIAMENT LIGHTS 100S
BENSON & HEDGES LIGHTS 100S	MERIT KING SIZE
BENSON & HEDGES ULTRA LIGHT 100S	CAMBRIDGE 100S
BENSON & HEDGES ULTRA LIGHT 100S BOX	NOW 100S
BENSON & HEDGES REGULAR SIZE BOX	NOW KING SIZE BOX
BULL DURHAM KING SIZE	OLD GOLD 100S
CAMBRIDGE 100S	NOW 100S
CAMBRIDGE KING SIZE	NOW KING SIZE BOX
CAMBRIDGE KING SIZE BOX	*QUIT*
CAMEL REGULAR SIZE NF	CAMEL KING SIZE
CAMEL KING SIZE	WINSTON LIGHTS 100S
CAMEL KING SIZE FILTER BOX	VICEROY KING SIZE
CAMEL LIGHTS 100S	MORE LIGHT 100S

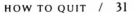

BRAND AND TYPE YOU SMOKE NOW	BRAND AND TYPE TO SWITCH TO
CAMEL LIGHTS KING SIZE	WINSTON ULTRA LIGHTS 100S
CAMEL LIGHTS KING SIZE BOX	WINSTON ULTRA LIGHTS 100S
CARLTON 120S	CARLTON 100S
CARLTON 100S	NOW 100S
CARLTON 100S BOX	NOW KING SIZE BOX
CARLTON KING SIZE	NOW KING SIZE BOX
CARLTON KING SIZE BOX	*QUIT*
CARLTON SLIMS 100S	CARLTON 100S
CENTURY 100S	KENT 100S
CENTURY KING SIZE	RALEIGH KING SIZE
CENTURY LIGHTS KING SIZE	WINSTON ULTRA LIGHTS 100S
CENTURY LIGHTS 100S	WINSTON LIGHTS 100S
CHESTERFIELD KING SIZE NF	WINSTON 100S
CHESTERFIELD REGULAR SIZE NF	VICEROY KING SIZE FILTER
DORAL II	NOW 100S
DORADO KING SIZE	VANTAGE KING SIZE
ENGLISH OVALS KING SIZE NF BOX	ENGLISH OVALS REGULAR SIZE NF BOX
ENGLISH OVALS REGULAR SIZE NF BOX	CAMEL REGULAR SIZE NF
EVE LIGHTS 120S	EVE LIGHTS 100S
EVE LIGHTS 100S	VANTAGE 100S
GALAXY KING SIZE	VANTAGE KING SIZE
HALF AND HALF KING SIZE	PALL MALL 100S FILTER
HERBERT TAREYTON KING SIZE NF	WINSTON 100S
KENT 100S	TRUE GOLD KING SIZE
KENT KING SIZE	KENT GOLDEN LIGHT KING SIZE
KENT KING SIZE BOX	KENT GOLDEN LIGHT KING SIZE
KENT GOLDEN LIGHTS 100S	TRUE 100S
KENT GOLDEN LIGHTS 100S BOX	WINSTON ULTRA LIGHTS 100S
KENT GOLDEN LIGHTS KING SIZE	PARLIAMENT LIGHTS KING SIZE
KENT GOLDEN LIGHTS KING SIZE BOX	WINSTON ULTRA LIGHTS 100S
KENT III 100S	KENT III KING SIZE
KENT III KING SIZE	BARCLAY KING SIZE
KENT III KING SIZE BOX	BARCLAY KING SIZE
L AND M 100S	MARLBORO LIGHTS 100S
L AND M KING SIZE	MARLBORO LIGHTS 100S
L AND M KING SIZE BOX	MARLBORO LIGHTS KING SIZE BOX

BRAND AND TYPE YOU SMOKE NOW	BRAND AND TYPE TO SWITCH TO
L AND M LIGHTS 100S	CARLTON 120S
L AND M LIGHTS KING SIZE	MERIT KING SIZE
LARK 100S	WINSTON LIGHTS 100S
LARK LIGHTS 100S	WINSTON LIGHTS 100S
LARK KING SIZE	L AND M LIGHTS KING SIZE
LARK LIGHTS KING SIZE	L AND M LIGHTS KING SIZE
LUCKY STRIKE REGULAR SIZE NF	PALL MALL KING SIZE
LUCKY STRIKE 100S	PALL MALL LIGHT 100S
LUCKY STRIKE KING SIZE	LUCKY STRIKE LIGHTS KING SIZE
LUCKY STRIKE KING SIZE BOX	LUCKY STRIKE LIGHTS KING SIZE
LUCKY STRIKE LIGHTS KING SIZE	MERIT KING SIZE
MAGNA KING SIZE	WINSTON LIGHTS 100S
MAGNA LITES KING SIZE	WINSTON LIGHTS KING SIZE
MARLBORO 100S	PARLIAMENT LIGHTS 100S
MARLBORO 100S BOX	PARLIAMENT LIGHTS 100S
MARLBORO 25S 100S	PARLIAMENT LIGHTS 100S
MARLBORO KING SIZE	MULTIFILTER KING SIZE
MARLBORO KING SIZE BOX	MULTIFILTER KING SIZE BOX
MARLBORO 25S KING SIZE	MULTIFILTER KING SIZE
MARLBORO LIGHTS 100S	PARLIAMENT LIGHTS KING SIZE
MARLBORO LIGHTS 100S BOX	PARLIAMENT LIGHTS KING SIZE BOX
MARLBORO LIGHTS KING SIZE	MERIT KING SIZE
MARLBORO LIGHTS KING SIZE BOX	MERIT KING SIZE
MAX 120S	WINSTON 100S
MERIT 100S	MERIT KING SIZE
MERIT KING SIZE	VANTAGE ULTRA LIGHTS KING SIZE
MERIT KING SIZE BOX	VANTAGE ULTRA LIGHTS 100S
MERIT ULTRA LIGHTS 100S	VANTAGE ULTRA LIGHTS 100S
MERIT ULTRA LIGHTS KING SIZE	TRUE KING SIZE
MORE 120S	MARLBORO 100S
MORE LIGHTS 100S	VANTAGE ULTRA LIGHTS 100S
MULTIFILTER KING SIZE	PARLIAMENT LIGHTS KING SIZE
NEWPORT RED KING SIZE	TRUE GOLD LIGHTS KING SIZE
NEWPORT RED KING SIZE BOX	VANTAGE KING SIZE
NOW 100S	NOW KING SIZE
NOW 100S BOX	NOW KING SIZE BOX
NOW KING SIZE	NOW KING SIZE BOX
NOW KING SIZE BOX	*QUIT*

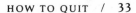

BRAND AND TYPE YOU SMOKE NOW	BRAND AND TYPE TO SWITCH TO
OLD GOLD STRAIGHT KING SIZE NF	OLD GOLD FILTER 100S
OLD GOLD KING SIZE	CAMEL KING SIZE
OLD GOLD FILTER 100S	OLD GOLD KING SIZE
OLD GOLD LIGHTS KING SIZE	TRUE 100S
PARLIAMENT LIGHTS 100S	PARLIAMENT LIGHTS KING SIZE
PARLIAMENT LIGHTS KING SIZE	MERIT KING SIZE
PARLIAMENT LIGHTS KING SIZE BOX	MERIT KING SIZE
PALL MALL KING SIZE NF	PALL MALL KING SIZE
PALL MALL 100S	TAREYTON 100S
PALL MALL KING SIZE	TAREYTON KING SIZE
PALL MALL LIGHT 100S	MERIT ULTRA LIGHTS 100S
PALL MALL EXTRA LIGHT KING SIZE	CARLTON 100S
PHILLIP MORRIS COMMANDER NF	PHILLIP MORRIS REGULAR SIZE NF
PHILLIP MORRIS REGULAR SIZE NF	BENSON & HEDGES 100S
PHILLIP MORRIS INTERNATIONAL BOX	TAREYTON 100S
PLAYERS REGULAR SIZE BOX NF	CAMEL REGULAR SIZE NF
PLAYERS 100S BOX	MERIT 100S
PLAYERS KING SIZE BOX	PARLIAMENT LIGHTS KING SIZE BOX
PLAYERS LIGHTS 100S 25S	VANTAGE 100S
PLAYERS LIGHTS KING SIZE 25S	PARLIAMENT LIGHTS KING SIZE
RALEIGH KING SIZE NF	WINSTON 100S
RALEIGH 100S	WINSTON LIGHTS 100S
RALEIGH KING SIZE	WINSTON LIGHTS KING SIZE
RALEIGH LIGHTS KING SIZE	CAMEL LIGHTS KING SIZE
RALEIGH LIGHTS 100S	MERIT KING SIZE
RICHLAND 100S	RALEIGH 100S
RICHLAND KING SIZE	VICEROY KING SIZE
RICHLAND LIGHTS 100S	RALEIGH LIGHTS 100S
RICHLAND LIGHTS KING SIZE	CAMEL LIGHTS KING SIZE
RITZ LOW TAR 100S	VICEROY RICH LIGHTS 100S
ST. MORITZ 100S	VICEROY RICH LIGHTS 100S
SARATOGA 120S	PALL MALL LIGHTS 100S
SATIN 100S	PALL MALL LIGHTS 100S
SILVA THINS 100S	PALL MALL LIGHTS 100S
STERLING KING SIZE BOX	MULTIFILTER KING SIZE
STERLING 100S BOX	PARLIAMENT LIGHTS 100S
STERLING KING SIZE	MULTIFILTER KING SIZE

BRAND AND TYPE YOU SMOKE NOW	BRAND AND TYPE TO SWITCH TO
TALL 120S	WINSTON 100S
TAREYTON 100S	MARLBORO LIGHTS 100S
TAREYTON KING SIZE	MARLBORO LIGHTS KING SIZE
TAREYTON LONG LIGHTS 100S	CARLTON 100S
TAREYTON LIGHTS KING SIZE	NOW 100S
TRIUMPH 100S	NOW 100S
TRIUMPH KING SIZE	NOW KING SIZE
TRUE 100S	WINSTON ULTRA LIGHT 100S
TRUE KING SIZE	KENT III KING SIZE
TRUE GOLD 100S	VANTAGE 100S
TRUE GOLD KING SIZE	PARLIAMENT LIGHTS KING SIZE
VANTAGE 100S	VANTAGE ULTRA LIGHT 100S
VANTAGE KING SIZE	VANTAGE ULTRA LIGHT 100S
VANTAGE ULTRA LIGHT 100S	VANTAGE ULTRA LIGHT KING SIZE
VANTAGE ULTRA LIGHT KING SIZE	NOW 100S
VICEROY SUPER LONGS 100S	WINSTON LIGHTS 100S
VICEROY KING SIZE	VICEROY RICH LIGHTS KING SIZE
VICEROY RICH LIGHTS 100S	MORE LIGHTS 100S
VICEROY RICH LIGHTS KING SIZE	MERIT KING SIZE
VIRGINIA SLIMS 120S	PARLIAMENT LIGHTS 100S
VIRGINIA SLIMS 100S	MERIT 100S
VIRGINIA SLIMS LIGHT 100S BOX	BENSON & HEDGES ULTRA LIGHT 100S BOX
WINSTON 100S	KENT 100S
WINSTON INTERNATIONAL 100S BOX	KENT KING SIZE
WINSTON KING SIZE	KENT KING SIZE
WINSTON KING SIZE BOX	KENT KING SIZE
WINSTON LIGHTS 100S	MORE LIGHTS 100S
WINSTON LIGHTS 100S BOX	WINSTON ULTRA LIGHTS 100S
WINSTON LIGHTS KING SIZE	WINSTON ULTRA LIGHTS 100S
WINSTON LIGHTS KING SIZE BOX	WINSTON ULTRA LIGHTS 100S
WINSTON ULTRA LIGHT 100S	VANTAGE ULTRA LIGHT KING SIZE
WINSTON ULTRA LIGHTS KING SIZE	NOW 100S

Source: Federal Trade Commission Report to Congress, January 1985

MASTER LIST

For Switching Down to a Lower Tar/Nicotine Level

MENTHOL CIGARETTES

HOW TO USE THE LIST

1. Find your brand and type in the left-hand column. Switch down to the brand in the right-hand column.
2. Switch to a new brand every three weeks.
3. Work your way down and off the list.
Very important! Do not substitute sizes or packages. Box and Soft Pack are almost always different strengths. King Size, 100s and 120s are almost always different strengths. If you can't find what you want, refer to the Do-It-Yourself chapter.

All brands are filter cigarettes unless marked "NF," Non-Filter.
All packages are Soft Packs unless marked "Box."

BRAND AND TYPE YOU SMOKE NOW	BRAND AND TYPE TO SWITCH TO
ALPINE KING SIZE	MERIT 100S
BARCLAY 100S	NOW 100S
BARCLAY KING SIZE	NOW KING SIZE
BELAIR KING SIZE	MERIT KING SIZE
BELAIR 100S	VANTAGE ULTRA LIGHTS 100S
BENSON & HEDGES 100S	MULTIFILTER KING SIZE
BENSON & HEDGES 100S BOX	MULTIFILTER KING SIZE
BENSON & HEDGES LIGHTS 100S	MERIT KING SIZE
BENSON & HEDGES ULTRA LIGHT 100S BOX	NOW 100S
BRIGHT 100S	NOW 100S
BRIGHT KING SIZE	NOW 100S
CARLTON 120S	CARLTON 100S
CARLTON 100S	NOW 100S
CARLTON 100S BOX	*QUIT*
CARLTON KING SIZE	*QUIT*
DORAL II KING SIZE	NOW 100S
EVE LIGHTS 120S BOX	EVE LIGHTS 100S
EVE LIGHTS 100S	BENSON & HEDGES LIGHTS 100S
ICEBERG 100S	BARCLAY KING SIZE

BRAND AND TYPE YOU SMOKE NOW	BRAND AND TYPE TO SWITCH TO
KENT 100S	BELAIR 100S
KENT GOLDEN LIGHTS 100S	BELAIR 100S
KENT GOLDEN LIGHTS KING SIZE	BELAIR 100S
KOOL REGULAR SIZE NF	KOOL KING SIZE FILTER
KOOL KING SIZE	KOOL MILD 100S
KOOL KING SIZE BOX	KOOL MILDS 100S
KOOL SUPER LONG 100S	KOOL LIGHTS 100S
KOOL MILDS 100S	SALEM LIGHTS 100S
KOOL MILDS KING SIZE	SALEM LIGHTS KING SIZE
KOOL MILDS KING SIZE BOX	SALEM LIGHTS KING SIZE
KOOL LIGHTS 100S	MERIT KING SIZE
KOOL LIGHTS KING SIZE	MERIT KING SIZE
KOOL ULTRA 100S**	CARLTON 100S
KOOL ULTRA KING SIZE**	SALEM ULTRA KING SIZE
LUCKY STRIKE 100S	LUCKY STRIKE LIGHTS 100S
LUCKY STRIKE KING SIZE	LUCKY STRIKE LIGHTS KING SIZE
LUCKY STRIKE LIGHTS KING SIZE	MERIT KING SIZE
MARLBORO KING SIZE	SALEM LIGHTS KING SIZE
MAX 120S	MORE 120S
MERIT 100S	MERIT KING SIZE
MERIT KING SIZE	MERIT ULTRA LIGHT KING SIZE
MERIT ULTRA LIGHTS 100S	NOW 100S
MERIT ULTRA LIGHTS KING SIZE	TRIUMPH KING SIZE
MONTCLAIR KING SIZE	SALEM LIGHTS KING SIZE
MORE 120S	KOOL MILDS 100S
MORE LIGHT 100S	VANTAGE ULTRA LIGHTS
MULTIFILTER KING SIZE	MORE LIGHTS 100S
NEWPORT 100S	NEWPORT KING SIZE
NEWPORT KING SIZE	NEWPORT LIGHTS 100S
NEWPORT KING SIZE BOX	NEWPORT LIGHTS 100S
NEWPORT LIGHTS 100S	MORE LIGHTS 100S
NEWPORT LIGHTS KING SIZE	MERIT KING SIZE
NEWPORT LIGHTS KING SIZE BOX	MERIT KING SIZE
NOW 100S	BARCLAY KING SIZE
NOW KING SIZE	CARLTON KING SIZE OR *QUIT*
PALL MALL LIGHT 100S	SALEM LIGHTS KING SIZE
PHILLIP MORRIS INTERNATIONAL 100S BOX	KOOL MILDS 100S

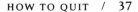

BRAND AND TYPE YOU SMOKE NOW	BRAND AND TYPE TO SWITCH TO
PLAYERS 100S BOX	MERIT 100S
PLAYERS KING SIZE BOX	MORE LIGHT 100S
PLAYERS LIGHTS 25S KING SIZE	MORE LIGHTS 100S
PLAYERS LIGHTS 25S, 100S	MORE LIGHTS 100S
RICHLAND KING SIZE	KOOL MILDS 100S
RITZ 100S	SALEM LIGHTS 100S
ST. MORITZ 100S	KOOL SUPER LONG 100S
SALEM KING SIZE	KOOL KING SIZE BOX
SALEM 100S	KOOL MILDS 100S
SALEM LIGHTS 100S	MORE LIGHTS 100S
SALEM SLIM LIGHTS 100S	BRIGHT 100S
SALEM LIGHTS KING SIZE	MORE LIGHTS 100S
SALEM ULTRA LIGHTS 100S	NOW 100S
SALEM ULTRA KING SIZE	TRIUMPH KING SIZE
SARATOGA 120S	BENSON & HEDGES LIGHTS 100S
SATIN 100S	MORE LIGHTS 100S
SILVA THINS 100S	BENSON & HEDGES LIGHT 100S
SPRING 100S	KOOL MILDS 100S
STERLING 100S BOX	MULTIFILTER KING SIZE
STERLING KING SIZE BOX	MULTIFILTER KING SIZE
TALL 120S	SALEM 100S
TRIUMPH 100S	TRIUMPH KING SIZE
TRIUMPH KING SIZE	BARCLAY KING SIZE
TRUE 100S	TRUE KING SIZE
TRUE KING SIZE	TRIUMPH KING SIZE
VANTAGE 100S	BRIGHT 100S
VANTAGE KING SIZE	MERIT KING SIZE
VANTAGE ULTRA LIGHTS 100S	NOW 100S
VANTAGE ULTRA LIGHTS KING SIZE	NOW 100S
VIRGINIA SLIMS 100S	BENSON & HEDGES LIGHT 100S
VIRGINIA SLIMS LIGHTS 100S BOX	MERIT KING SIZE

**Do not switch to any size or package of Kool Ultra or Kool Ultra 100s.
Source: Federal Trade Commission Report to Congress, Janauary 1985.

THE MOST DIFFICULT TIME

I can predict the most difficult time you will experience while you are quitting, and why it occurs. Sometimes it helps to know what to expect and to remember that any pangs that you may suffer will really be very minimal in comparison to what you would experience if you simply tried to give up cigarettes all at once. I guarantee that there will be no comparison at all to that awful agony.

You may experience two kinds of minor discomfort. One of these is called "taste discomfort" and the other "nicotine discomfort" and they are due to entirely different causes.

Taste Discomfort

The first kind of discomfort you may suffer is taste discomfort. Here is how it will work.

Let us say that our typical smoker is using Marlboro King Size cigarettes in a soft pack. This brand and type is the most popular brand and type of cigarettes sold in the United States today. According to the FTC, Marlboro has a tar content of 16 milligrams per cigarette. If, by switching to another brand, you drop 3 milligrams of tar it means you are dropping 19 percent with the switch. I was told that double blind product testing indicated that this amount of change is noticeable and disliked by only 7 percent of respondents. After one week, the percentage of respondents calling the change noticeable and disliked dropped to 4 percent. So the chances that it will cause you trouble are minimal. At this level, I can almost promise you that any discomfort will be gone in only a few days.

Taste differences will become more noticeable each time that you switch when you get down to cigarettes that have 4 milligrams of tar and less. For example, let us say you are dropping from a Now 100 Soft Pack at 3 milligrams tar to a New King Size Soft Pack at 1 milligram tar. This means that you are dropping the tar content, or taste value, of your cigarette by 67 percent. You are cutting your tar consumption by two-thirds. This will be noticeable; it may be irritating for a few days, and it may be somewhat frustrating. But **just keep smoking** the lower tar/nicotine, cigarette. Smoke as many as you need to. You will be very happy with them in less than a week and your smoking will return to its normal pattern.

Again, testing showed that at such a low level of tar consumption, any discomfort passed quickly. In one week, less than 5 percent of smokers noticed any change at all at this level.

Well, you say. Why don't you switch me to a regular cigarette with only 2 mg tar—and make my life easier with a drop of only 33 percent?

That is easy to answer. I would if I could. There are no regular-tasting cigarettes with 2 milligrams tar.

There is one other kind of taste discomfort that you may notice when you shift between different kinds of taste. I have been told that additives and taste enhancement are more frequently used by American Tobacco Company brands. If you switch to an R.J. Reynolds brand that uses less taste enhancers, you may notice a difference. You may or may not like the difference initially, but within a few days you shouldn't notice it at all. Also, if you switch to or from a charcoal-filter cigarette, you may notice a taste change that you may not like. Just remember:

- In most cases, it will pass in a week.

- It is part of the unavoidable price of changing brands.

- In three weeks you will be switching to another brand and type anyway, so bear with it.

- If you really cannot stand it, go to the do-it-yourself section of the book; look up the cigarette you do not like in the left hand column; pick another brand and type with the **same** nicotine content and try that brand and type.

Nicotine Discomfort

Everything that has been said about taste discomfort is almost exactly the same for nicotine discomfort.

If you are smoking a Marlboro King Size Soft Pack at 1.0 milligrams nicotine and you drop to Multifilter King Size Soft Pack at 0.8 milligrams, you are cutting your nicotine intake by 0.2 milligrams per cigarette, or 20 percent.

When you get down to the lower-nicotine cigarettes the situation is different. For example, you may be dropping from a Now King Size Box at .05 milligrams to a Carlton King Size Box at .01 milligrams. This cuts your nicotine intake by 5, or 80 percent. Even though it is a very small drop, it will be noticeable because it is such a big percentage drop. By the same token, however, the frustration will not be as bad as it sounds because your nicotine addiction is already at a very low level. All I can suggest is that you bear with it for a couple of days (that is all it should take) until any frustration goes away. Meanwhile just smoke more cigarettes until your body gets used to being addicted at a lower level.

THE FINAL STEP: QUITTING

As soon as you are comfortable with Carlton King Size Box, you should try to quit smoking entirely. By this time, your addiction level should be so low that you can smoke or not smoke, as you desire, **as long as you never smoke anything stronger than a Carlton King Size Box cigarette.**

I gave up cigarettes before my husband did. He continued smoking Carlton King Size Box. Knowing the harm he could do to himself, I objected to his smoking anything at all. At that time he was under a huge business strain and he just couldn't give them up. So we compromised. When he worked, he smoked; but he never smoked at night, on weekends, or during vacation. To the best of our knowledge, at least from what we recall, neither one of us had any difficulty with this arrangement. Now, thank God, we both have stopped smoking altogether.

I cannot tell you that quitting, which is your last step, will take place without some frustration. But I do know that if, for example, you are smoking Carlton King Size Box, the pangs will be only 1 percent of what they would have been had you tried to quit with a Marlboro King Size addiction. So you will have saved yourself 99 percent of the pain.

One of the respondents after trying the system said that it "wasn't any worse than giving up chocolate."

I don't believe that, and you probably won't either; but at any rate, it will be 99 times easier than it would be for a Marlboro smoker.

CHAPTER FIVE

Tricks & Traps

W hen I read what I have written, I am sometimes afraid that it sounds as if the cigarette companies are all in a conspiracy to keep smokers addicted. That is not true. There is no conspiracy.

They simply know their business. They have a lot of money, which you give them every day. They know that smokers are addicted, they hire the very best product, marketing and advertising people around and they spend enormous sums on advertising, promotion and consumer research to keep them smoking. They all follow basically the same strategy for only one reason: **It works.**

Their managements know all the tricks of the marketing trade. They will give away free cigarettes, free lighters, big coupon price discounts, whatever they can think of or whatever they have to do to keep you hooked on their brand. They will run beautiful four-color six-page spreads in a dozen magazines to attract smokers and to convince them to use, or keep using, their products. They will put on rock and jazz concerts and sponsor tennis challenge cups to get your good will. They have huge war chests for their lobbyists and they will avidly contribute to the reelection campaigns of any politician who will support their cause.

They are pros. They are very well paid, and they should be because they run very big businesses. For example, it is easy to figure out from the company's 1985 annual report that Brown and Williamson's profit on the Kool brand alone was over $300 million in that one year. That's right. **Three hundred million dollars profit** on just that one brand in only one year. That is not gross. I mean **profit.** And Kool is a small brand. It is not one of the big sellers like Marlboro, Winston, Merits or Benson & Hedges. That is why the management and the research people at the tobacco companies are so good. Most are graduates of Procter and Gamble, General Foods, Kellogg or other highly professional marketing/ brand management organizations. Once they are acquainted with the fundamentals of the tobacco business, it is not difficult for them to design the basis of a product/marketing strategy that will keep a smoker addicted.

Let's see, how do I describe how they do it.

The way we are taught to describe something is research, you should always start with the most general aspect, what is sometimes called the "big picture," and then work down to the specifics of what you are trying to say. Well, how the cigarette companies describe their brands is the most general thing I can think of right now, so I shall start there.

HOW THE CIGARETTE INDUSTRY DESCRIBES ITS BRANDS

The first thing you have to know is how they trick and trap you about what you **think** you are smoking. So what I am going to do is show you what you **are** smoking—and that when you think you are smoking a "Low Tar Cigarette" you are probably **not doing any such thing.** It is just one of the small ways the cigarette manufacturers fool you into happily smoking a higher tar/nicotine brand than you might think you are smoking.

I will explain. Since most people think that the terms "Regular Strength," "Low Tar," and "Ultra Low Tar" are governement-regulated descriptions of cigarette strength, I am going to tell you, right off, that it is just not so. The government has **nothing** to do with these descriptions.

Are you surprised at that?

I was.

I thought that those terms were established according to government guidelines.

Not so at all. And when I learned that from the FTC, don't you think I felt stupid, especially after all the cigarette studies I have done.

The terms are simply non-binding, broad, industry descriptions of cigarette classes. They have been carefully crafted to deceive the smoker about what he is smoking. Now I will tell you what they really mean, and why they are structured the way they are.

When the Surgeon General brought out his first report in 1963, it caused a lot of people to become more concerned about smoking cigarettes than they had ever been before. The industry calls these people the "health concerned" segment of the market. Naturally, they wanted to sell to these people, so they developed new versions of their products that they called Lights or Low Tar cigarettes, like Marlboro Lights. At this point they were faced with a problem. Regular strength cigarettes were 15 milligrams tar and they didn't want too much of a gap between their regular cigarettes and the new Low Tar versions because people would become dissatisfied and switch to another brand. So they brought out the new versions of their brands at 12 milligrams. Testing showed that a difference this size would not cause people to become dissatisfied and switch.

However, from a health standpoint, 12 milligrams isn't really a low tar cigarette. It is fully 75 percent as strong as a regular cigarette. As the public's concern about cigarettes heightened, more and more milder brands were brought out. Today, with the increased emphasis on health, three out of four brands are below 12 milligrams. The industry still calls them "Low Tar," but at 80 percent of full strength, they are still very strong cigarettes.

Why is this important? It is important because the cigarette companies use the descriptions to make smokers think that they are protecting themselves by smoking a low tar cigarette when actually they are not doing anything of the kind. In short, a low tar cigarette is not low in tar. If anything, it should be called a medium tar cigarette. What the industry calls an ultra low tar cigarette is not ultra low in tar. It is really just plain low in tar.

When you look at the industry classifications given below, they may seem perfectly reasonable at first glance. But when you look at them carefully, you will see that low tar, or lights, are almost as strong as a regular cigarette.

CIGARETTE CLASSIFICATIONS

Industry Description	Tar Range	Should Be Called
Regular Strength	16 to 12 mg	High Tar
Low Tar or Lights	12–6 mg	Medium Tar
Ultra Low Tar	Under 6 Mg	Low Tar

The tobacco companies have set their standards for a low tar cigarette so high for only one reason: to make smokers think they are smoking a low tar cigarette when they are really smoking a medium tar cigarette. They don't want a smoker to be concerned about what he is smoking, so they set the standards for calling a cigarette low tar as high as possible so that more brands fall within the standard. Smokers who use these brands feel safer, but they are really smoking a cigarette that is 75 percent as strong as the strongest of the popular cigarettes, and they don't know it.

Who can really blame the poor smoker for not knowing what he or she is smoking. People who smoke cannot be expected to understand all of the intricacies with which the cigarette companies describe their brands in relation to the structure of the market. They know cigarettes are dangerous and the government monitors tar and nicotine levels, so smokers naturally assume that the government sets the standards as well.

Also, since the designation of Lights or Low Tar is strictly informal, companies can and do violate it. For example, Eve Light 120s, regular and menthol, are 14 milligrams tar and 1.0 milligram nicotine, or stronger than a Kent 100 and as strong as an L & M 100 and a Newport Red. Yet they call it a Light and indeed they can because **they make their own rules.**

What applies to the Low Tar classification also applies to the industry classification of Ultra Low Tar cigarettes. Any cigarette under 6 milligrams is called an Ultra Low Tar by the cigarette makers, when it should really be called a Low Tar cigarette. Why should it only be called Low Tar? Because it occupies the lower one-third of a high, medium and low tar classification system for filter cigarettes. It is almost exactly one-third of the way down the scale from 0 to 16 milligrams.

Again, the cigarette companies have deliberately created their industry definitions to make the smokers think they are smoking something safer than they are really smoking. The whole purpose of this exercise is the same as the "Low Tar/Lights" idea—to keep smokers unworried, while keeping their level of addiction as high as possible. The message is simple:

DON'T PAY ATTENTION TO THE INDUSTRY DEFINITIONS. THEY ARE DELIBERATELY SET HIGHER TO MAKE YOU THINK YOU ARE SMOKING A SAFER CIGARETTE—WHEN YOU PROBABLY ARE NOT DOING ANYTHING OF THE KIND.

All right, you ask. How can I know what I am smoking?

Of course, you should be paying attention to the list of switching instructions in Chapter 4. If that does not work for you, or if you want to design your own quitting program, pay careful attention to the tar/nicotine levels themselves in Chapter Six, the do-it-yourself section of this book.

That is not as easy as you think. Either way you choose, you will have to proceed carefully because the companies have laid every kind of a product/marketing trap that they can think of in order to keep you smoking a higher tar cigarette. Read on.

Why the Tobacco Companies Hide the Tar/Nicotine Levels

You realize, of course, that you should be paying attention to the tar/nicotine levels. But where does the average smoker like yourself find the figures for each brand's tar/nicotine level when the cigarette companies try to hide the truth from you. They are not given on the package.

We have given the FTC tar/nicotine figures in Chapter 6 of this book. But where else could you possibly find them? The newspapers haven't published the figures since January of 1985, because the FTC has stopped publishing them. According to what I read in the *New York Times,* this was done to satisfy the objections of the "Tobacco Senators." They said it was "undue publicity" and if anyone wanted to know what they were, they could write to the FTC for the information.

But now the FTC won't give them out. How do I know? I called the FTC and tried to get their updates for this book. According to Ms. Judith Wilkrenfeld at the FTC (telephone (202) 326-3150), the agency is **still doing the testing, but will no longer release the figures to Congress or to the public.**

THE ONLY PLACE YOU CAN FIND THE FIGURES FOR TAR AND
NICOTINE LEVELS IS IN THIS BOOK.

It gets worse.

Saying it is unfair discrimination against the tobacco industry to
have the figures published, the Tobacco Senators are now attempting to get the FTC to stop testing altogether. After all, they argue,
why should the federal government single out the tobacco industry
for this kind of discriminatory public testing any more than the
vegetable industry or the fruit industry or any other section of the
economy.

At this point, the smoker who wants to quit would have to
search the magazine advertisements to try to find out what cigarette
has a lower tar and nicotine level than the one he or she is smoking.
Who in the world is going to do that?

How Cigarette Manufacturers Use the
Length of a Cigarette to Confuse Smokers

Many years ago the cigarette companies found that most smokers
thought a longer cigarette was milder because the extra length
filtered the smoke more before it got to their lungs.

Aha, the cigarette marketers said. Here we added 20 percent to
the tar and nicotine in a cigarette and people think it is milder. So
their next step was to do some research on the meaning of mildness.
They found out what any smoker knows already. A milder-tasting
cigarette **means** a lower-tar cigarette to a smoker, and therefore a
safer, less dangerous cigarette to smoke. That is not necessarily true.
You can easily make a stronger, milder-tasting cigarette by using
more Virginia tobacco and less Burley in the blend. The English do
this all the time and it is why English cigarettes taste different from
American cigarettes. But the important thing is that smokers **think**
it is true, because any salesman will tell you that, in selling, per-
ception is more important than reality.

So what did the cigarette companies do with this information?
They did what any sane and sensible marketer would do. They gave
the smokers what they wanted. They gave them longer cigarettes
and they put on massive advertising campaigns calling the new
cigarettes—you guessed it—**milder.**

And it was very successful.

Is that the only thing they do with size? No, it is not.

Sometimes they really do give the longer version of a brand the same or lower tar/nicotine count. So you have to be careful about cigarette lengths, and be sure to smoke **exactly** the size and type and package as it is given on the list.

Here is a comparison of the nicotine content in two different sizes for three brands of cigarettes. Notice that the first cigarette has up to 6 times more nicotine than the second cigarette, which is simply a different size. This illustrates why you have to be so careful when trying to switch brands and types of cigarettes in order to really get a cigarette with lower nicotine.

NICOTINE LEVELS BY BRAND SIZE

Brand and Size	Nicotine Level (mg)
Carlton 120	.6
Carlton King Size	.1
True 100	.7
True King Size	.4
Now 100	.3
Now King Size	.1

Source: FTC Report, January 1985

Let the novice beware. The Carlton King Size smoker, who is trying to cut down, could pick up a Carlton 120 and say "My, isn't this a satisfying version of a Carlton. I think I will switch to this," not realizing that it is **6 times stronger.** Of course, the smoker is better satisfied. The poor guy is floating up there on a nicotine high. A couple of packs and he or she is hooked again at a higher level and will be wondering why in the world it is so hard to switch down the next time he or she is supposed to go to a lower level of addiction. Switching down is definitely not easy, the person will say. Not so. The smoker has been tricked because he was not **careful.** You will have to watch every detail if the system of switching down is to work.

How Cigarette Manufacturers Use the Package to Confuse Smokers

But there is an even more important way that the cigarette makers try to confuse the smoker. They use the package.

The cigarette marketers know that people were switching down and out on their own. They also knew that once smokers get down to 1 or 2 milligrams of tar and 0.1 or 0.2 milligrams of nicotine it is easy for them to quit smoking.

A friend of mine who did a lot of research for one of the other major cigarette companies said he knew it because they did a tracking study for them. They first used psychographics to isolate the Health Concerned smoker. Then, knowing who they were, they isolated that segment of the Health Concerned market who smoked high tar/nicotine brands, figuring that a good proportion of them would start switching down, which proved to be the case. They tracked everybody's habits, right down to Carlton Box and Now Box. Eighty-one percent of those who got to 1 milligram tar (.1 milligram nicotine) quit. If they got down as far as the box, over 90 percent quit. The study also showed that most people think all packages of a brand are the same strength, that is that all Marlboro boxes are the same strength, all Winston soft packs are the same, and all Carlton boxes are the same strength. So they confused the packages.

Here is what he meant by "confusing the packages." Since both of the big manufacturers of low-tar cigarettes do essentially the same thing, they confuse a high proportion of smokers into smoking something higher than what they think they are smoking. You can see the strategy in simple form in this comparison of nicotine variation by the kind of package bought.

Brand and Package	Amount of Nicotine
Carlton 100s Box	.1 mg
Carlton 100s Soft Pack	.4 mg

Source: FTC Report, January 1985

Look at the two figures. Carlton 100 soft pack is **4 times** as strong as Carlton 100 Box. The same brand, the same length, a different package and a totally different level of nicotine addiction for the unwary smoker who does not ask carefully enough for the correct package. That is why smokers who are trying to switch down and wean themselves away from higher tar/nicotine brands must order exactly and precisely what the list tells them to order. Otherwise the cigarette companies will bounce the smoker right back up to a higher nicotine level and an addiction that is just as bad, or perhaps worse, than before switching. Someone who had made this mistake would find it hard to drop further; without knowing it, the smoker went back up to a .4 or a .6 addiction level instead of a .1 level.

Here is what R.J. Reynolds does with Now box. It is really the same story as Carlton but with a different package, and the differences are not as extreme:

Brand and Package	Amount of Nicotine
Now 100s Box	.1 mg
Now 100s Soft Pack	.3 mg

Source: FTC Report, January 1985

So there you have it again. R.J. Reynolds is doing exactly the same thing with the Now 100 Box and soft pack packages that the American Tobacco is doing with their Carlton packages. Now 100s Box is three times as strong as Now 100s Softpack.

The lessons:
- FOLLOW THE INSTRUCTIONS CAREFULLY.
- DO NOT ACCEPT SUBSTITUTES.
- ORDER BY THE CARTON TO INSURE A SAFE SUPPLY.
- NEVER, NEVER TRADE UP.

Tricks with Filters and Fingers

There are a number of other ways that the cigarette companies try to keep your addiction higher. Since you should be aware of what they are, I am going to tell you about them, but I also want to say to you, right off, that in many cases there is really not much that you or any smoker can do to protect yourself from them, except in the case of Barclay, Kool Ultra and Kool Ultra 100s. **Do not smoke** those brands. I will tell you why below.

There are four ways that cigarette manufacturers reduce the tar/nicotine levels in their brands. First, as we have already discussed, they use reconstituted tobacco. The second means is the cigarette paper. They use a more porous paper in the lower tar brands and a less porous paper in the higher tar brands. Since more porous paper lets in more air as a person inhales, it reduces the amount of smoke and therefore the tar/nicotine that a person inhales.

The third means of creating a lower tar/nicotine cigarette is the filter. They simply make a more effective filter, one that lets less tar pass through and thus creates a lower tar cigarette. Actually, all the hullabaloo about filters is vastly overrated, since the cigarette companies, as you would expect if you think about it, can easily make a filter that is 100 percent effective. No smoke would get through at all. The only problem with this idea is that the tar creates the taste. So, if you really clean up the smoke, you will have a cigarette with no tar (taste) and no nicotine (addiction satisfaction).

To a cigarette company, filters are just marketing tools. Design a filter that is different and that the smoker thinks is more effective and you may have a sales advantage among smokers who fall into the Health Concerned classification.

The fourth way that the companies reduce the tar/nicotine levels is by adding air holes or vents to let in air, dilute the smoke and thereby create a lower-tar product. They work in much the same way as the porous paper and usually they are placed on the filter tip. Actually, they serve three purposes:

1. They reduce the tar/nicotine counts in the FTC tests.

2. They can be advertised to lull smokers into thinking they are smoking a safer "air-filtered" cigarette (or some other such nonsense).

3. They are placed at positions on the tip, where they will reduce tar/nicotine in an FTC test, **but will be covered up by the smokers' lips or fingers as they inhale.**

What this means, of course, is that low-tar smokers are always smoking a somewhat higher level of nicotine and tar and therefore staying addicted at a higher level than they think that they really are. The diagrams show how it works.

There really is not very much any smoker can do about this

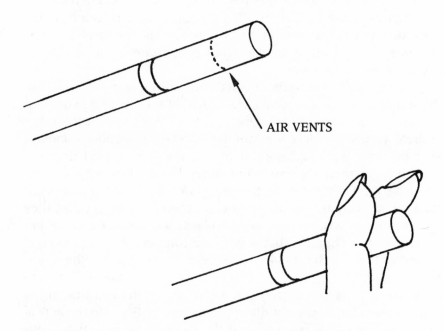

AIR VENTS

kind of description because it is impossible to think about what you are doing every puff that you take. (Figuring 15 puffs to the cigarette, the two-pack-a-day smoker takes about 350 puffs a day.)

The best example I know of what they can do with vents is what Brown and Williamson did with Barclay cigarettes. It was so outrageous that even the other cigarette companies put in a complaint to the FTC about Barclay, which is something that they very seldom do about a competitor. It was so bad, the FTC finally took them to court—and won.

Here is what the Barclay filter looked like from an end view.

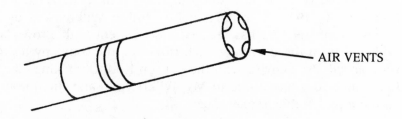

AIR VENTS

This filter perfectly satisfies the FTC tests as a 1 miligram tar and .1 milligram nicotine cigarette. That is because the FTC test machine does **not** crush the end of the cigarette. But smokers are **not** machines, and when a smoker smokes a cigarette, his lips automatically crush the vents.

When the air vents are crushed, the smoke is not diluted and the smoker ends up smoking a cigarette that is estimated to be from 3 to 7 milligrams tar (FTC Report, 1984). This angered the other cigarette companies since it meant that Barclay would addict smokers at a nicotine level higher than they could match, and that any smoker who tried Barclay could never be satisfied with a competitive Ultra Light cigarette. Brown and Williamson stood to eventually steal away the whole Ultra Light market. With Barclay, they violated the unwritten industry standards we described in the beginning of this chapter. That is why the competitors complained.

According to the 1984 FTC Report to Congress, "the Commission successfully sued ... enjoin Brown and Williamson from advertising its Barclay cigarette as a 1 mg tar cigarette or from using any tar number not specifically approved by the FTC." In the appeal of that decision, the court upheld the FTC's contention that "consumers do rely on the ratings to make comparative assessment of the adverse health effects of cigarettes; that Barclay cigarettes deliver disproportionately more tar than other similarly rated cigarettes; and that disclaimers in advertising to explain the difference will prove ineffective."

The FTC Report of January 1984 goes on to state "that there was a signficant likelihood that the same problem (namely, an inaccurate reporting of the "tar," nicotine and CO delivery) existed with respect to Kool Ultra and Kool Ultra 100s, two other brands manufactured by Brown and Williamson."

In other words, Brown and Williamson figured out how to pull the wool over the FTC's eyes, using the FTC's own tests. It was not until the other cigarette companies complained that an embarassed FTC sued successfully and stopped them from advertising. As of February 20, 1986, according to Ms. Judith Wilkrenson, of the Commission, the FTC has reached a settlement with Brown and Williamson on the Barclay matter. However, the company has not yet reached a settlement with the FTC on Kool Ultra King Size, or Kool Ultra 100s, according to Ms. Wilkrenson, and the questions on these two brands remain open.

Because of the FTC cautionary note, I would advise that smokers wishing to quit by switching down SHOULD STAY CLEAR of both of the two Brown and Williamson brands under challenge. Do not switch to any size or package of Kool Ultra or Kool Ultra 100s.

Regular and Menthol

One of the most interesting findings of cigarette consumer research is that many smokers believe that menthol cigarettes are less dangerous than regular-tasting cigarettes. This is somehow related to the menthol taste, which masks the strength of the tobacco smoke by creating a sensation of coolness in the mouth. This leads many smokers to feel that menthol cigarettes are somehow milder and therefore less dangerous to smoke.

This is not so. The menthol-flavored versions of cigarette brands are sometimes stronger, sometimes milder and sometimes exactly the same strength as the regular-tasting version. In this way, the smoker can easily be confused into smoking a higher-strength cigarette. That is why I keep repeating, if you want to switch down and out, be very careful about what you buy and do not assume **anything,** because they are deliberately trying to confuse you.

In the table below we give examples of three brands and their menthol and regular cigarette tar/nicotine strengths; one set is higher, one set is lower, and one set is the same. Read them and

TAR/NICOTINE LEVEL
Regular- and Menthol-Flavored Brands

Brand and Type	Tar	Nicotine
Menthol Higher Strength		
Now 100s Regular Box	*	.1 mg
Now 100s Menthol	3 mg	.3 mg
Menthol Lower Strength		
Carlton 100s Regular	5 mg	.4 mg
Carlton 100s Menthol	1 mg	.1 mg
Menthol the Same Strength		
Vantage 100s Regular	9 mg	.7 mg
Vantage 100s Menthol	9 mg	.7 mg

*So low, it's not measurable.
Source: FTC Report, January 1985

beware. Now Menthol 100s are three times stronger than Now 100s Regular!! Carlton 100s Regular have four times as much nicotine as Carlton 100s Menthol. That's right, **4 times** stronger. That is why we tell you to be careful. If you don't watch out you will get zapped.

Name Confusion

One company even uses the descriptions on the package to confuse the smoker. This only occurs in one instance, and in one brand, Kools, so I am not making a big point of it. However, I do think that it should be mentioned so that you will not be caught in case you are smoking Kools.

What they have done is create a new classification called "Milds" as opposed to Lights and made this classification somewhat stronger than Lights. If the poor smoker who is smoking Lights switches to Milds, he is immediately bounced up to a greater tar/nicotine level. (see the comparison below).

Brand and Type	Tar	Nicotine
Kool Lights King Size	8 mg	0.7*
Kool Milds King Size Box	12 mg	1.0**
Kool Lights 100S	9 mg	0.7*

*Source: FTC Report, January 1985
**Source: Manufacturer's Advertisement

I know many smokers have been fooled; as one respondent told me, "I took your advice. Now I smoke Kool Milds. They're one of the lowest tar cigarettes you can buy."

Nonsense. Kool Milds King Size Box, have 12 milligrams of tar and 1.0 mg of nicotine. They are **over 40 percent stronger** in nicotine than either Kool Lights King Size or Kool Lights 100s. That is why I keep emphasizing how careful you have to be in order to drop your addiction to a point low enough to quit. My husband and I fought the frustration and the desire for another cigarette for much too long, and we know how hard it is.

Do It Yourself

The purpose of this chapter is to help you design a do-it-yourself program for switching brands to get a steadily lower tar/nicotine level each time. Despite all my efforts to make things easier by taking into account taste, tar levels, nicotine levels and image, my suggestions simply may not meet your needs. You may end up hating the taste of something that I have picked.

In that case, you can use the lists below to help yourself out by selecting a brand and type that suits you better. Or maybe developing your own tailor-made system for reducing tar/nicotine levels is a better solution for you and your particular needs. In doing this, you can use trial and error or whatever other means you wish to choose brands that satisfy your nicotine habit while you keep cutting your intake.

Giving you the facts gives you complete flexibility, and some people enjoy that. Like David Riesman's "inner-directed" people, they love doing everything themselves. One of us is like that; my husband believes that people will do better in an atmosphere of complete freedom where they have the responsibility to do what is best for themselves. So in this book you have your choice of the best of both worlds, or any combination thereof. You can rely on us, you can do it yourself, or both.

Before you start off on a do-it-yourself program, I would like to give you a little information that I think may make your choices easier.

Most cigarette brands are only slightly different in their ranking by their tar or nicotine content, since when a cigarette company reduces one component, it usually automatically reduces the other. However, you will notice from the FTC values that follow that there is a considerable difference from cigarette to cigarette in the **way** tar and nicotine levels drop, because the manufacturers have sometimes taken special steps to reduce one factor to a greater extent than the other. I suggest that you pay more attention to the nicotine content, since it is nicotine that creates the addiction and therefore the frustration.

This is not to underestimate the importance of taste, but simply to say that it is not the factor that causes addiction. Most smokers trying to quit would rather live with less taste than more frustration. For this reason, the brands are listed in descending order by their nicotine content, rather than by their tar content. This is also the way that the FTC ranks the brands in its report.

NINE IMPORTANT SUGGESTIONS

Here are nine important suggestions, based on years of research among smokers like you.

1. Please be very careful about cigarette size and type of package. As I explained in the chapter on tricks and traps, this is one of the main ways cigarette companies will trap you into smoking a stronger cigarette and a higher addiction level.

2. Do not try to quit any faster than you feel comfortable with. If you wait until you are completely satisfied with each change, you will probably avoid a build-up of frustration.

3. If you are now smoking a regular-strength cigarette, (1.0 to 2.1 milligrams nicotine), I suggest that you drop at the rate of .3 milligrams of nicotine and 3 milligrams of tar at a time until you reach 1.0 milligrams nicotine.

4. After 1.0 milligrams nicotine, drop .2 milligrams of nico-tine at a time until you get to .4 milligrams of nicotine. When you get to .4 milligrams of nicotine, drop by only .1 milligrams nicotine at a time.

5. When you reach the .1 milligrams level of nicotine, and are comfortable at this level, switch to "Now" King Size Box until you are ready to quit. Be very careful about "Now" cigarette sizes and box types. The "Now" 100 Box is twice as strong as the "Now" King Size Box.

6. Buy your cigarettes by the carton so that you will not run out of the brand to which you have switched down.

7. Do not let storekeepers tell you they have stopped manu-facturing a brand. It is their favorite cop-out. Find some-one who will special order what you want.

8. And most important: **Never, never trade up, even for one cigarette.**

9. If you need to buy or borrow a stronger cigarette don't be embarrassed. Take a pencil and punch holes between the filter and the tobacco to weaken the smoke.

Here is the ranking of cigarette brands and types as published by the FTC. For convenience' sake, and also to avoid confusion between different variations of the same brand I have reorganized these into two lists, one for regular and one for menthol cigarettes, to make it easier for you. The first list gives the strengths of regular cigarettes and the second list contains the information on menthol cigarettes.

Each list is organized from the strongest to the weakest brand and type of cigarette. You will be working your way **down** the list. You will find your brand and type of cigarette in the left-hand column and you should start from there. Choose the cigarette you want to switch down to, keeping in mind my suggestions 3, 4 and 5 as to the amount of drop to select.

Good luck and success.

TAR AND NICOTINE CONTENT
Regular Cigarette Brands

All packages are Soft Pack unless marked "box."
All cigarettes are filter unless marked NF, Non-Filter.

		CONTENT	
BRAND NAME	**TYPE**	**Nicotine** *(Mg)*	**Tar** *(Mg)*
ENGLISH OVALS	KING SIZE BOX NF	2.1	28
PLAYERS	REG SIZE BOX NF	1.9	25
BULL DURHAM	KING SIZE	1.8	28
ENGLISH OVALS	REG SIZE BOX NF	1.8	23
PHILLIP MORRIS COMMANDER	KING SIZE NF	1.6	26
OLD GOLD STRAIGHT	KING SIZE NF	1.6	26
HERBERT TAREYTON	KING SIZE NF	1.5	24
CHESTERFIELD	KING SIZE NF	1.5	22
TALL 120S	120 MM	1.5	20
OLD GOLD FILTER 100S	100 MM	1.5	20
RALEIGH	KING SIZE NF	1.4	25
LUCKY STRIKE	REG SIZE NF	1.4	23
CAMEL	REG SIZE NF	1.4	21
MAX 120S	120 MM	1.4	18
PALL MALL	KING SIZE NF	1.3	23
HALF & HALF	KING SIZE	1.3	18
RICHLAND 100S	100 MM	1.3	17
MORE 120S	120 MM	1.3	17
OLD GOLD FILTER	KING SIZE	1.3	17
PHILLIP MORRIS	REG SIZE NF	1.2	21
CHESTERFIELD	REG SIZE NF	1.2	19
WINSTON 100S	100 MM	1.2	17
CENTURY 100S	100 MM	1.2	17
RICHLAND	KING SIZE	1.2	17
WINSTON	KING SIZE	1.2	16
PHILLIP MORRIS INTERNATIONAL	100 MM	1.1	17
PALL MALL	KING SIZE	1.1	17
WINSTON INTERNATIONAL 100S	100 MM BOX	1.1	16
WINSTON	KING SIZE BOX	1.1	16
CAMEL FILTER	KING SIZE BOX	1.1	16

BRAND NAME	TYPE	CONTENT	
		Nicotine *(Mg)*	Tar *(Mg)*
PALL MALL 100S	100 MM	1.1	15
CENTURY	KING SIZE	1.1	15
BENSON & HEDGES	KING SIZE BOX	1.1	15
ST. MORITZ 100S	100 MM	1.1	14
EVE LIGHTS 120S	120 MM	1.1	14
RALEIGH 100S	100 MM	1.0	16
CAMEL FILTER	KING SIZE	1.0	16
CAMEL FILTER	KING SIZE BOX	1.0	16
MARLBORO 100S	100 MM	1.0	16
MARLBORO 25 100S	100 MM	1.0	16
MARLBORO 100S	100 MM BOX	1.0	16
MARLBORO	KING SIZE	1.0	16
MARLBORO 25	KING SIZE	1.0	16
MARLBORO	KING SIZE BOX	1.0	16
BENSON & HEDGES 100S	100 MM	1.0	16
BENSON & HEDGES 100S	100 MM BOX	1.0	16
LARK 100S	100 MM	1.0	15
VIRGINIA SLIMS 120S	120 MM	1.0	14
MAGNA	KING SIZE	1.0	14
NEWPORT RED	KING SIZE	1.0	14
L & M 100S	100 MM	1.0	14
LARK LIGHTS 100S	100 MM	1.0	13
RITZ	100 MM·BOX	1.0	13
KENT 100S	100 MM	1.0	13
STERLING	100 MM BOX	1.0	12
STERLING	KING SIZE BOX	1.0	12
VICEROY	KING SIZE	0.9	16
RALEIGH	KING SIZE	0.9	15
VIRGINIA SLIMS 100S	100 MM	0.9	14
SARATOGA 120S	120 MM BOX	0.9	14
LARK	KING SIZE	0.9	14
GALAXY	KING SIZE	0.9	14
VICEROY SUPERLONG 100S	100 MM	0.9	14
TAREYTON 100S	100 MM	0.9	13
TAREYTON	KING SIZE	0.9	13
DORADO	KING SIZE	0.9	13
LARK LIGHTS	KING SIZE	0.9	13
KENT	KING SIZE BOX	0.9	12

| BRAND NAME | TYPE | CONTENT | |
		Nicotine (Mg)	Tar (Mg)
L & M	KING SIZE	0.9	13
L & M	KING SIZE BOX	0.9	13
PLAYERS LIGHTS 100S	100 MM	0.9	12
NEWPORT RED	KING SIZE BOX	0.9	12
CENTURY LIGHT 100S	100 MM	0.9	12
KENT	KING SIZE	0.9	12
KENT	KING SIZE BOX	0.9	12
CAMEL LIGHTS 100S	100 MM	0.9	12
EVE LIGHTS 100S	100 MM	0.9	12
RICHLAND LIGHTS 100S	100 MM	0.9	11
SILVA THINS 100S	100 MM	0.9	11
TRUE GOLD 100S	100 MM	0.9	11
LUCKY STRIKE 100S	100 MM	0.9	11
SATIN 100S	100 MM	0.9	10
PLAYERS LIGHTS	KING SIZE BOX	0.8	12
PARLIAMENT LIGHTS 100S	100 MM	0.8	12
MULTIFILTER	KING SIZE	0.8	12
CAMEL LIGHTS 100S	100 MM	0.8	11
WINSTON LIGHTS 100S	100 MM	0.8	11
VICEROY RICH LIGHTS 100S	100 MM	0.8	11
LUCKY STRIKE	KING SIZE BOX	0.8	11
MARLBORO LIGHTS	100 MM BOX	0.8	11
RICHLAND LIGHTS	KING SIZE	0.8	10
CENTURY LIGHT	KING SIZE	0.8	10
PLAYERS LIGHTS 25S	KING SIZE	0.8	10
RALEIGH LIGHTS	KING SIZE	0.8	10
LUCKY STRIKE	KING SIZE	0.8	10
TRUE GOLD	KING SIZE	0.8	10
OLD GOLD LIGHTS	KING SIZE	0.8	9
KENT GOLDEN LIGHTS 100S	100 MM	0.8	9
KENT GOLDEN LIGHTS	KING SIZE	0.8	9
L & M LIGHTS 100S	100 MM	0.8	8
WINSTON LIGHTS	KING SIZE BOX	0.7	11
VICEROY RICH LIGHTS	KING SIZE	0.7	10
MERIT 100S	100 MM	0.7	10
MARLBORO LIGHTS 100S	100 MM	0.7	10
MARLBORO LIGHTS 100S BOX	100 MM	0.7	10

BRAND NAME	TYPE	CONTENT	
		Nicotine *(Mg)*	Tar *(Mg)*
MARLBORO LIGHTS	KING SIZE	0.7	10
MARLBORO LIGHTS	KING SIZE BOX	0.7	10
BENSON & HEDGES LIGHTS 100S	100 MM	0.7	10
WINSTON LIGHT 100S	100 MM BOX	0.7	9
VANTAGE 100S	100 MM	0.7	9
VANTAGE	KING SIZE	0.7	9
RALEIGH LIGHTS 100S	100 MM	0.7	9
CENTURY LIGHTS	KING SIZE	0.7	9
PALL MALL LIGHT 100S	100 MM	0.7	9
CAMEL LIGHTS	KING SIZE BOX	0.7	9
KENT GOLDEN LIGHTS 100S	100 MM BOX	0.7	8
KENT GOLDEN LIGHTS	KING SIZE BOX	0.7	8
WINSTON LIGHTS	KING SIZE	0.7	8
LUCKY STRIKE LIGHTS	KING SIZE	0.7	8
L & M LIGHTS	KING SIZE	0.7	8
TRUE 100S	100 MM	0.7	7
PARLIAMENT LIGHTS	KING SIZE	0.6	9
PARLIAMENT LIGHTS	KING SIZE BOX	0.6	9
MAGNA LIGHTS	KING SIZE	0.6	9
CAMEL LIGHTS	KING SIZE	0.6	9
MORE LIGHTS 100S	100 MM	0.6	8
VIRGINIA SLIMS LIGHTS	100 MM BOX	0.6	8
CARLTON 120S	120 MM	0.6	7
TAREYTON LONG LIGHTS	100 MM	0.6	7
PALL MALL EXTRA LIGHT	KING SIZE	0.6	7
CARLTON SLIMS	100 MM	0.6	6
BENSON & HEDGES ULTRA LIGHTS	100 MM	0.6	6
MERIT ULTRA LIGHTS 100S	100 MM	0.6	6
MERIT	KING SIZE BOX	0.5	8
MERIT	KING SIZE	0.5	8
WINSTON ULTRA LIGHTS 100S	100 MM	0.5	5
VANTAGE ULTRA LIGHTS 100S	100 MM	0.5	5
MERIT ULTRA LIGHTS	KING SIZE	0.5	5
BARCLAY	100 MM	0.4	5
WINSTON ULTRA LIGHTS	KING SIZE	0.4	5

BRAND NAME	TYPE	CONTENT	
		Nicotine *(Mg)*	Tar *(Mg)*
VANTAGE ULTRA LIGHTS	KING SIZE	0.4	5
KENT III	100 MM	0.4	5
BENSON & HEDGES ULTRA LIGHT	100 MM BOX	0.4	5
CARLTON 100S	100 MM	0.4	5
CAMBRIDGE 100S	100 MM	0.4	5
TRUE	KING SIZE	0.4	4
TRIUMPH 100S	100 MM	0.4	4
TAREYTON LIGHTS	KING SIZE	0.4	4
DORAL II	KING SIZE	0.4	4
TRIUMPH	KING SIZE	0.3	3
NOW 100S	100 MM	0.3	3
KENT III	KING SIZE	0.3	3
KENT III	KING SIZE BOX	0.3	3
BARCLAY	KING SIZE	0.2	3
BARCLAY	KING SIZE BOX	0.2	3
NOW	100 MM BOX	0.1	1
CARLTON 100S	100 MM BOX	0.1	1
NOW	KING SIZE	0.1	1
CAMBRIDGE	KING SIZE	0.1	1
BENSON & HEDGES	REG SIZE BOX	0.1	1
CAMBRIDGE	KING SIZE BOX	0.05	.5
NOW	KING SIZE BOX	0.05	.5
CARLTON	KING SIZE BOX	0.05	.5

Source: Federal Trade Commission Report, January 1985, plus updates from advertisements and the cigarette companies where available.

TAR AND NICOTINE CONTENT
Menthol Cigarette Brands

All packages are Soft Pack unless marked "box."
All cigarettes are filter unless marked NF, Non-Filter.

BRAND NAME	TYPE	CONTENT	
		Nicotine *(Mg)*	Tar *(Mg)*
NEWPORT 100S	100 MM	1.5	19
MAX 120S	120 MM	1.4	19
TALL 120S	120 MM	1.3	17
KOOL	REGULAR SIZE NF	1.2	20
RICHLAND	KING SIZE	1.2	18
NEWPORT	KING SIZE	1.2	17
SALEM 100S	100 MM	1.2	16
MORE 120S	120 MM	1.2	16
KENT 100S	100 MM	1.2	15
SPRING 100S	100 MM	1.1	19
PHILLIP MORRIS INTERNATIONAL	100 MM	1.1	17
NEWPORT	KING SIZE BOX	1.1	16
SALEM	KING SIZE	1.1	16
KOOL	KING SIZE BOX	1.1	16
EVE LIGHTS 120S	120 MM BOX	1.1	14
ST MORITZ 100S	100 MM	1.1	14
MARLBORO	KING SIZE	1.0	16
KOOL	KING SIZE	1.0	16
BENSON & HEDGES 100S	100 MM	1.0	16
BENSON & HEDGES 100S	100 MM BOX	1.0	16
MONTCLAIR	KING SIZE	1.0	15
RITZ	100 MM BOX	1.0	13
LUCKY STRIKE 100S	100 MM	1.0	12
LUCKY STRIKE	KING SIZE	1.0	12
KOOL MILDS	KING SIZE BOX	1.0	12
STERLING	100 MM	1.0	12
STERLING	KING SIZE	1.0	12
PALL MALL LIGHT 100S	100 MM	1.0	12
ALPINE	KING SIZE	0.9	16
VIRGINIA SLIMS 100S	100 MM	0.9	14
KOOLS SUPER LONG 100S	100 MM	0.9	14

BRAND NAME	TYPE	CONTENT	
		Nicotine *(Mg)*	Tar *(Mg)*
SARATOGA 120S	120 MM BOX	0.9	14
PLAYERS 100S	100 MM	0.9	13
PLAYERS LIGHTS 100S 25S	100 MM BOX	0.9	13
EVE LIGHTS 100S	100 MM	0.9	12
KOOL MILDS 100S	100 MM	0.9	12
KOOL MILDS	KING SIZE	0.9	12
SILVA THIN 100S	100 MM	0.9	11
MULTIFILTER	KING SIZE	0.8	12
PLAYERS	KING SIZE BOX	0.8	12
PLAYERS LIGHTS	KING SIZE	0.8	12
NEWPORT LIGHTS 100S	100 MM	0.8	10
SALEM LIGHTS 100S	100 MM	0.8	10
SALEM LIGHTS	KING SIZE	0.8	10
SATIN 100S	100 MM	0.8	9
KENT GOLDEN LIGHTS 100S	100 MM	0.8	9
KENT 100S	100 MM	0.8	9
BENSON & HEDGES LIGHTS 100S	100 MM	0.7	10
BELAIR	KING SIZE	0.7	10
VANTAGE 100S	100 MM	0.7	9
VANTAGE	KING SIZE	0.7	9
MERIT 100S	100 MM	0.7	9
KOOL LIGHTS 100S	100 MM	0.7	9
NEWPORT LIGHTS	KING SIZE BOX	0.7	9
LUCKY STRIKE LIGHTS	KING SIZE	0.7	8
NEWPORT LIGHTS	KING SIZE	0.7	8
KENT GOLDEN LIGHTS	KING SIZE	0.8	9
SALEM SLIM LIGHTS 100S	100 MM	0.7	8
KOOL LIGHTS	KING SIZE	0.7	8
TRUE 100S	100 MM	0.7	7
VIRGINIA SLIM LIGHTS	100 MM BOX	0.6	8
MORE LIGHT 100S	100 MM	0.6	8
BELAIR 100S	100 MM	0.6	8
CARLTON 120S	120 MM	0.6	7
MERIT	KING SIZE	0.5	8
KOOL ULTRA 100S	100 MM	0.5	6
KOOL ULTRA	KING SIZE	0.5	6
BRIGHT 100S	100 MM	0.5	6

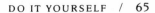

BRAND NAME	TYPE	CONTENT	
		Nicotine *(Mg)*	Tar *(Mg)*
BRIGHT	KING SIZE	0.5	6
VANTAGE ULTRA LIGHTS 100S	100 MM	0.4	5
VANTAGE ULTRA LIGHTS	KING SIZE	0.4	5
CARLTON 100S	100 MM	0.4	5
TRUE	KING SIZE	0.4	5
SALEM ULTRA LIGHTS 100S	100 MM	0.4	5
SALEM ULTRA LIGHTS	KING SIZE	0.4	5
BARCLAY 100S	100 MM	0.4	5
BENSON & HEDGES ULTRA LIGHT BOX	100 MM	0.4	5
MERIT ULTRA LIGHTS	KING SIZE	0.4	5
MERIT ULTRA LIGHTS 100S	100 MM	0.4	4
TRIUMPH 100S	100 MM	0.4	4
DORAL II	KING SIZE	0.4	4
ICEBERG 100S	100 MM	0.3	4
TRIUMPH	KING SIZE	0.3	3
NOW 100S	100 MM	0.2	2
BARCLAY	KING SIZE	0.2	3
KOOL ULTRA**	KING SIZE	0.2	3
NOW	KING SIZE	0.1	1
CARLTON	KING SIZE	0.1	1
CARLTON 100S	100 MM BOX	0.05	0.5

**Do not switch to any size or package of Kool Ultra or Kool Ultra 100s.*

Source: Federal Trade Commission Report To Congress, January 1985, plus updates from advertisements and the cigarette companies where possible.

The Dangers of Smoking

N ot even the cigarette companies bother to deny that cigarette smoking is dangerous anymore. I recently read about a lawsuit brought against R.J. Reynolds by the family of a smoker who had died of lung cancer. The company structured a large part of its defense on the proposition that smokers are warned about the dangers of smoking cigarettes. They said that the warnings are right on the package and that R.J. Reynolds does not claim cigarette smoking is not dangerous. Both the jury and the appeals courts have upheld the company's argument as valid.

The Surgeon General has now written about ten reports since 1963. You may not realize how much data is available, but these reports are based on the life records of millions and millions of people who have been tracked by the government for over 30 to 40 years. In this chapter I quote primarily from three American studies in the Surgeon General's Reports to Congress of 1980, 1982, and 1984.*

---

*Data on health hazards of smoking are contained in several of the Surgeon General's Reports to Congress. See 1980; Smoking and Health; 1982; Smoking and Cancer; 1983; Smoking and Cardio-Vascular Disease; 1984; Smoking and Chronic Obstructive Lung Disease (COLD); and 1985; Cancer and Chronic Lung Disease in the Workplace. The data discussed in this chapter is derived mainly from three large American datasets that constitute the principal statistical under-pinnings of these reports. One of these datasets exists as a study in itself, the Veterans' Study. The other two datasets are derived from a 25-state study conducted by the American Cancer Society. This results in more uniform data since it reduces the number of variables in data development.

In this chapter, I primarily quote from two big studies in the Surgeon General's reports to Congress. I didn't choose these at random. First, I selected large studies because big studies are so much more likely to be accurate and reliable. Second, I wanted American studies, because this book is primarily written for Americans, and studies about your own people are always going to mean more to you than studies about people in a foreign place, no matter how accurate the foreign studies may be.

ACCURACY OF THE ODDS
Studies in the Surgeon General's Reports to Congress*

Name of Study Reported	Sample Size	Minimum Accuracy	Reliability
Veterans	290,000	1/9th of 1%	95% Level of Confidence
ACS**—Men	358,000	1/10th of 1%	95% Level of Confidence
ACS**—Women	483,000	1/11th of 1%	95% Level of Confidence

*Refers only to the Surgeon General's Report on Smoking for the years of 1980, 1982, 1983, 1984.
**American Cancer Society

What all that statistical jargon means is that 95% of the time, any of the numbers in this chapter are going to be correct within about one tenth of one percent (999 times out of 1,000).

So many studies have been conducted that they would fill several long library shelves. In addition to the ones I quote, the Surgeon General has other American studies and huge studies from England, Sweden, Japan and other countries where there is socialized medicine. In these countries the government health departments keep long-term records on almost the whole country. This means that they can do studies on the long-term effects of cigarettes much more easily than we can here in the United States. As a person who is familiar with research statistics, I can tell you that when the numbers are this big, and they come in from all over the world showing exactly the same pattern of findings, the results are really irrefutable.

All of these studies prove, beyond any measure of doubt, that cigarette smoking is a cause of cancer, heart disease, emphysema, cardiovascular illness, fetal injury, premature birth, low birth weight and other problems. The list is long enough and the facts are ghoulish enough to scare almost anyone.

The reports consistently show that cigarette smokers die at a younger age than nonsmokers: cancer, emphysema, heart attack; all are ugly ways to die.

In addition, if smoking doesn't kill you, it will inevitably affect your lifestyle and keep you from doing the kinds of things you would like to do. Sports are, of course, the activity most affected by smoking cigarettes. They damage your ability to breathe and therefore your strength and your stamina. The carbon monoxide deprives your brain of oxygen and slows your reaction time. The reports prove this; and slow mental reactions do not help you in business, either. The reports are engorged with facts, because with numbers of this size almost any effect on a person or a lifestyle can be measured.

When I talk with people, however, I am surprised to find that most of the facts are not very well known. On second thought, it is not really so surprising. The newspapers and television only give you a quick summary of the most dramatic (not necessarily the most important) findings in each report. Then the report quickly becomes yesterday's news and it is shelved away in the government documents room at your local library. No one but an occasional researcher putters in there to read the facts. When I went to our local library at Post College in Nassau County, New York, in the course of my research some of the copies of the Surgeon General's Report hadn't been pulled in over two years.

Here are some of the facts.

CANCER

The Surgeon General's reports show that cigarettes are a cause of early death from cancer. Like most people, I knew that cigarette smoking would cause cancer in many people. That was not news to me. What really did make me sit up and pay attention to what I thought would be a long, dull report was the number of **kinds** of cancer that cigarette smoking is associated with. So many kinds of cancer the media doesn't have time to tell people about all of them. That was a shock to me. I had always though of cigarettes as causing lung cancer, but I had never given much thought to the connection between cigarettes and other kinds of cancer.

How the Odds Are Quoted

Throughout this chapter, I quote the death rates in "odds" rather than percentages. That is because I think that almost everyone is familiar with the idea of "odds" for or against something. Since we are a nation of bettors on everything from horseraces to football games, it seems an easier way for people to understand statistics. I have learned from hard experience presenting hundreds of research reports that percentages are pretty obscure to a lot of people. As any consumer research director knows, a lot of top corporation executives have trouble understanding percentages.

If you are a smoker instead of a nonsmoker, the reports give the odds that you will die from some of the different kinds of cancer. Here is what caught my attention.

Mortality Rates for Smokers

Men cigarette smokers on average are 11 to 1 more likely to die from lung cancer than nonsmoking males. Women cigarette smokers are 4.4 to 1 more likely to die from lung cancer than nonsmoking women. In fact, the death rates for most kinds of cancers are greater for men who smoke than for women cigarette smokers. This is true for cancer of the mouth and throat and esophagus (6.4 to 1 more likely than a nonsmoker for men; 3.3 to 1 for women). Bladder cancer and pancreatic cancer death rates are also higher for male cigarette smokers than they are for women smokers.

Now, these figures make it appear as if it is less dangerous for women to smoke than it is for men to smoke. Actually, that is only partly true. In the past, women smokers have had better survival odds than men in comparison with nonsmokers of their sex for two reasons: they used to start smoking at an older age, and they used to smoke somewhat less than men. This meant that they did not take as much nicotine and tar into their systems. However, that is not true any longer. In today's world, women's smoking habits are much more similar to men's. The more recent data on younger women shows much the same pattern as younger men, with the result that only among older women smokers is the likelihood of death farther off.

The fact is that anyone who smokes cigarettes is more likely to die from cancer, and I mean many, many different kinds of cancer, than a nonsmoker.

Take a look at the table below.

ODDS A SMOKER IS MORE LIKELY
TO DIE OF CANCER THAN A NONSMOKER

Type of Cancer	Men Smokers	Women Smokers
Throat (Pharynx)	14.1 (to 1)	NA
Vocal Chords (Larynx)	11.5	NA
Lung	11.3	4.4 (to 1)
Mouth	6.5	NA
Esophagus only	6.4	4.9
Bladder	2.8	2.6
Pancreas	2.1	1.4
Stomach Cancer	1.5	1.3
Kidney Cancer	1.4	NA
Prostate	1.3	NA
Uterus	NA	1.2

Source: 1982 Surgeon General's Report on Smoking and Cancer, Part II.
NA: Not Applicable or Not Available

Also, when you look at all these odds, it is important to remember that these figures are for the average smoker. The more you smoke and the longer you have smoked, the higher your chances of dying from cancer; the less you smoke, the lower your chances. For example, as the next section shows, heavy smokers are about 25 times more likely to die from lung cancer than nonsmokers.

Lung Cancer

The Surgeon General's report specifically states that "cigarette smoking is the major cause of lung cancer in the United States. Smokers who consume two or more packs of cigarettes daily have lung cancer mortality rates 15 to 24 (23.7) times greater than nonsmokers." That is pretty clear. Now, let's look at some of the details.

Here are some of the ways of stating the odds that a veteran who smokes will die from lung cancer. If you smoke more than two packs a day, your odds of dying from lung cancer are 23.7 times greater than for a nonsmoker. If you smoke one to two packs a day, the odds are 16.7 times greater than for a nonsmoker, and if you smoke a half a pack to one pack a day they are 9.6 times greater. Now, to me these figures are enough to give a person nightmares. Before I did my research, I thought that the odds of dying would be, maybe, 3 or 4 to one. But 24 times as great? I mean **24 times** as great? That's like holding a loaded gun to your head.

However, the most frightening fact revealed by the data is how **little** you have to smoke to greatly increase your chances of dying from lung cancer. Even if you smoke less than half a pack a day, you are still 3.9 times as likely to get lung cancer as a nonsmoker (and my husband could never smoke as little as a half a pack a day; when he smoked, it was two packs a day or. more). The table below shows how quickly the odds go up as your smoking increases.

ODDS OF DYING FROM LUNG CANCER

Number of Cigarettes Smoked Each Day	Odds a Smoker Is More Likely to Die of Lung Cancer Than a Nonsmoker
1–9	3.9 (to 1)
10–20	9.6
21–39	16.7
40 or More	23.7

Source: 1982 Surgeon General's Report on Smoking and Cancer

Cancer of the Voice Box (Larynx)

Death rates are much higher for veterans who are heavy smokers. In fact, if a veteran smokes more than two packs a day, his death rate from cancer of the larynx was 34.4 times as great as for a nonsmoker: 17.2 times as great as a nonsmoker if he smoked one to two packs a day. Those figures are so awesome, I think I will stop right there. The following table shows all the figures for various degrees of smoking. Read them and weep.

ODDS OF DYING FROM CANCER OF THE LARYNX

Number of Cigarettes Smoked Each Day	Odds a Smoker Is More Likely to Die of Voice Box Cancer Than a Nonsmoker
1-10	4.4 (to 1)
11-20	13.5
21-40	17.2
Over 40	34.4

Source: 1982 Surgeon General's Report

Cancer of the Esophagus

If you don't know what your esophagus is, it is the tube between your throat and your stomach, the one the food gets stuck in when you swallow too much peanut butter sandwich at one time. Mortality rates for cancer of the esophagus among veterans are dramatically higher for heavy smokers. Veterans who smoked one to two packs of cigarettes a day are 12.4 times as likely to die of cancer of the esophagus as nonsmokers, as compared to odds of 3.1 to 1 if a smoker used less than half a pack a day. This means that the more cigarettes a smoker uses, the greater his chance of dying from this disease.

ODDS OF DYING FROM ESOPHAGEAL CANCER

Number of Cigarettes Smoked Each Day	Odds a Smoker Is More Likely to Die of Esophageal Cancer Than a Nonsmoker
1-9	3.1 (to 1)
10-20	4.3
21-39	12.4
40 or More	9.2

Source: 1982 Surgeon General's Report

In this table, there is a decline in the comparative death rate among smokers of two packs a day or more. It is not explained in the Surgeon General's report. It could be a statistical fluke due to the way the death rates were analysed, or it could be a real decline. But I would not want to use it as an excuse to smoke two packs a day or more.

Incidentally, unlike lung cancer, which is curable in some cases, the death rate from cancer of the throat and esophagus is 100%. That means everybody.

Bladder Cancer

Evidence of the effect of smoking on death rates from bladder cancer is shown in the table below. Taken from a study of 290,000 veterans, it shows that the more cigarettes they smoked, the greater their odds of dying from bladder cancer in comparison with a nonsmoker. The odds rise from 1.2 to 1 at half a pack a day or less to 2.8 to 1 against the smoker who is using one to two packs a day.

As an old friend of ours said when she read the first draft of the book: "It's another example of 'the more you use cigarettes, the quicker you go up in smoke.'" Then she laughed uproariously at her humor. I find it hard to laugh off numbers like these.

ODDS OF DYING FROM BLADDER CANCER

Number of Cigarettes Smoked Each Day	Odds a Smoker Is More Likely to Die of Bladder Cancer Than a Nonsmoker
1–9	1.2 (to 1)
10–20	2.2
21–39	2.8
40 or More	2.3

Source: 1982 Surgeon General's Report

Cancer of the Pancreas

There is no cure for pancreatic cancer.

The results of these studies show that men cigarette smokers are 2.1 times more likely to die from pancreatic cancer than non-smokers. Women cigarette smokers are 1.4 times as likely to die from cancer of the pancreas. Those are the odds for everybody. Here are the odds, depending on how much a person happens to smoke each day.

A study among 290,000 veterans showed that the more one smokes, the more likely one is to die from cancer of the pancreas. For example, if a veteran smokes less than 10 cigarettes per day, his chances of dying from pancreatic cancer are 1.6 times greater than a nonsmoker. These odds jump to 2.2 times as great for dying if the veteran smokes two packs a day or more. If you look at the figures in the table below, you will see that the death rate steadily increases with the number of cigarettes the smoker uses.

ODDS OF DYING FROM PANCREATIC CANCER

Number of Cigarettes Smoked Each Day	Odds a Smoker Is More Likely to Die of Pancreatic Cancer Than a Nonsmoker
1–9	1.6 (to 1)
10–20	1.7
21–39	2.0
40 or More	2.2

Source: 1983 Surgeon General's Report

HEART DISEASE

Subsequent research and analyses have resulted in similar findings about heart disease. The 1980 Surgeon General's report states, "Cigarette smoking is a major cause of coronary heart disease in the United States for both men and women. It should be considered the most important known modifiable risk factor." This means that if you quit, you stand a better chance of living.

The conclusion goes on to state: "Those who consume two or more packs a day have coronary heart disease death rates two and three times greater than nonsmokers." Since most people smoke a pack a day or more, the actual odds are 2.5 to 2. Note the table below:

ODDS OF DYING FROM HEART DISEASE

Number of Cigarettes Smoked Each Day	Odds a Smoker Is More Likely to Die of Heart Disease Than a Nonsmoker
All Smokers	2.5 (to 1)
Under 1 Pack	1.9
Over 1 Pack	2.6

Source: 1983 Surgeon General's Report

There are sound medical reasons for this cause and effect. One of the most frequent causes of heart attacks is that the arteries that feed the heart become clogged and close up. When this happens the part of the heart that they nourish dies: The heart stutters or stops, depending on how much of it is affected. In other words the person has a heart attack, and maybe dies.

Physiologically, nicotine has two primary effects on the heart. First, according to the 1983 Surgeon General's Report, smoking speeds up the "resting heartbeat by 15 to 25 beats per minute," which may be why so many people need a cigarette to get going in the morning. Second, it constricts the blood vessels, which is why your hands and feet get colder after a few cigarettes. This constricting of the blood vessels is the main reason that cigarette smoking is so bad for a person's heart. As the heart speeds up from the cigarette, the arteries are artificially and unnecessarily constricted, and there is a tendency for partially clogged arteries to close up. If that happens to one of the arteries feeding the heart, the person has a heart attack, or in that lovely euphemism of the medical profession, a "coronary accident."

Finally, according to the Surgeon General's Report in 1983, smoking boosts blood pressure by an average of 10 to 20 mmHg systolic and 5 to 15 mmHg diastolic. Obviously, higher blood pressure does not do a person any good either (except for the rare smoker who happens to have abnormally low blood pressure).

For us, the problem of heart attacks is even more personal because the odds are heavily weighted against the early-middle-aged smoker. The report shows that cigarette smokers in the 45-to-54-year-old age group are running a risk 7.0 times greater than nonsmokers of dying from heart attacks. The figures are not as dramatic as those for lung cancer, but they are still loaded against the smoker. Seven to 1 odds are still 7 to 1 odds against you if you smoke, and 45 to 54 is still a relatively young age to die from a heart attack by anyone's standards.

I had not expected that the odds of death from heart attacks would be dramatically worse for younger smokers than they are for older smokers. My expectation was that the older you were, the greater the risk would be to your heart if you smoked. In fact, the odds are over 5 times greater for smokers in the 45-to-54 age group than for smokers aged 75 to 84.

What does this mean? It means that you should be careful. If you are in the 45-to-54 age group, or younger, and you even suspect you have a heart problem, of if your parents or your grandparents have any history of heart problems, you had better quit smoking—fast—or nature might show you how to quit—the hard way. Note the odds below:

ODDS OF DYING FROM HEART DISEASE BY AGE

Age of Smoker	Odds a Smoker Is More Likely to Die of Heart Disease Than a Nonsmoker
45–54	7.0 (to 1)
55–64	1.8
65–74	1.6
75–84	1.2

Source: 1982 Surgeon General's Report, Table 9

These figures strike home to me in a very personal way. I have a son-in-law who is thirty-four and smokes. Now, his father and every male member of his father's family and his father have died of heart attacks when they were between the ages of 50 and 55. It's been true for three generations, and they were all smokers. Now, he should quit. He really should. He will not. With all the numbers pointing at him, he still laughs at the idea that the same thing will happen again. But my business is statistics, which means I get paid to figure the odds. When I consider how predisposed his family is to dying from heart attacks and that he smokes two packs a day, I conclude that the odds against him are a lot worse than 7 to 1.

And he has an adoring wife and three little children, two girls and a boy. His death would be an anguishing loss to his whole family.

Heart attacks are not pleasant. At best, they devastate your life; at worst, they kill you. Most people do not know this, but one third of the people who have a heart attack die with the first attack. Another third die with their second attack, and less than 2 percent survive the third heart attack. That is true even if you do not smoke.

Heart attacks are like playing Russian roulette with a three-chambered gun.

EMPHYSEMA AND BRONCHITIS

Emphysema is the big killer here. The odds are 14.2 to 1 times greater that a smoker will die from the disease than a nonsmoker. Emphysema is a prime example of a disease caused almost entirely by cigarettes. It was practically unknown before there was heavy cigarette smoking. With emphysema, you slowly suffocate because the cigarette smoke destroys your lungs. We have all seen people walking around dragging a portable oxygen tank behind them like a suitcase. That is because they have emphysema and their lungs are so debilitated that they can't get enough oxygen from the air.

The damage is caused by the tar in the cigarette smoke. What is generally called "tar" is actually a complex mixture of chemicals and acids, none of which are beneficial. For example, the "bite" that a cigarette produces in the back of a smoker's throat or lungs is largely caused, I am told, by chemical irritants, aldehydes and ketones, contained in the smoke. Since Burley tobacco is very rich in these chemicals, their "bite" (I used to kind of like it) restricts the amount of Burley that can be used in cigarettes (manufacturers like to use Burley because it is stronger tasting and less expensive than other types of tobacco).

However, the worst effects of tar are in the lungs themselves. When it gets to the lungs, the tar slowly clogs and burns the alveoli that the body uses to exchange fresh oxygen for waste carbon dioxide. As the alveoli become damaged, they can no longer exchange oxygen for carbon dioxide. When this happens to enough of the lungs, the smoker gets short of breath and eventually starts to turn blue and slowly suffocate. But since the process is gradual, the smoker really has had emphysema long before going to the doctor with a complaint.

Also, emphysema does not get better because the body cannot grow new oxygen-processing alveoli any more than it can grow new fingers or toes. What this means is that emphysema is incurable. It can be treated by drugs and oxygen, but it cannot be cured.

It only gets worse. Here are the figures for emphysema and bronchitis, with which more people are more familiar. The odds for bronchitis are not quite as bad as those for emphysema, only 4.5 to 1 against the smoker.

EMPHYSEMA AND BRONCHITIS MORTALITY RATES

Disease	Odds a Smoker Is More Likely to Die Than a Nonsmoker
Emphysema	14.2 (to 1)
Bronchitis	4.5

Source: 1984 Surgeon General's Report

CIGARETTE SMOKING AND PREGNANCY

There is factual evidence in the 1980 Surgeon General's Report that smoking cigarettes has a harmful effect on the fetus and on the health of a newborn baby.

The odds are 1.7 to 1 that a cigarette-smoking pregnant woman will have a spontaneous abortion, 1.4 times as great that she will have a premature baby. The odds are 2 to 1 that her baby will weigh less than a nonsmoker's baby. The baby of a cigarette smoking mother has a 1.3 times greater chance of being born dead or dying soon after birth (neonatal death). What wants to hurt babies? Note the table below.

ODDS OF PREGNANCY PROBLEMS

Type of Problem	Odds That Women Who Smoke Have Pregnancy Problems More Than Nonsmokers
Low Birth Weight	2.0 (to 1)
Spontaneous Abortion	1.7
Premature Baby	1.4
Fetal and/or Neonatal Death	1.3

Source: Surgeon General's 12th Annual Report, The Health Consequences of Smoking for Women. Bonhyam, G.S. and R.W. Wilson. "Children's health in families with cigarette smokers," American Journal of Public Health, March 1981.

THROMBOANGITIS OBLITERANS

Obliterans means that those who get the disease lose their fingers and toes because it obliterates their arteries. This disease, also called Buerger's disease, usually affects people of Russian or Polish extraction who are heavy smokers.

What happens is that a tobacco allergy causes blood clots to form on the linings of medium-sized arteries in the fingers and toes. This gradually blocks the arteries, causing painful ulcerations as the tissues die from gangrene. If the patient stops smoking, the tissues will heal quickly: If smoking is resumed, the ulcers reappear and the gangrene resumes until the fingers and toes have to be amputated.

However, if you do not have any Russian or Polish ancestry, you probably do not have to worry too much about this one, even if you smoke two packs a day or more.

TIME LOST

The National Center for Health Statistics records show that cigarette smokers, even in the comparatively young age group of 20 to 44, have to spend an extra 2.5 days in bed each year because of illness, as compared with nonsmokers. I was a little shocked at that figure because of how young the men who suffered most are. I had always thought of the bad effects of smoking as something that affects old men, and that a man could quit before it really hurt him.

Not so. Younger and very old men smokers spend more time sick in bed compared with middle-aged smokers. It is the other way around with women smokers. It hits middle-aged women smokers the hardest, comparatively.

DAYS OF BED DISABILITY PER YEAR

Age & Sex	Smoker	Nonsmoker	Difference
Men			
20–44	5.9	3.4	2.5
45–64	7.3	6.9	.4
65+	11.5	7.2	4.3
Women			
20–44	7.5	6.7	.8
45–64	11.5	8.3	2.2
65+	11.8	11.3	.5

Source: Smoking, Tobacco and Health, A Fact Book; US Department of Health and Human Services, Public Health Service, Office of Smoking and Health. Statistics quoted are from the National Center for Health Statistics.

Another set of figures, this time describing the association of smoking and chronic illness, shows that the odds are 1.7 to 1 greater that male smokers, age 20 to 44, will have limitations on their physical activity than nonsmokers. Again, it is the younger smokers who are getting hit the hardest in this data. It was another surprise for me. It is easy to see old men having the highest rates of chronic illness, but young guys, 20 to 44? That is something that I never expected—but there is the data and there is precious little anyone can do to deny it.

ODDS THAT CIGARETTE SMOKERS HAVE CHRONIC ILLNESS MORE OFTEN THAN A NONSMOKER

Men

20–44 years old	1.7 (to 1)
45–64 years old	1.1

Women

20–44 years old	1.3
45–64 years old	1.2

Source: 1980 Surgeon General's Report

Together, these two sets of figures show that smoking hurts a smoker at work and it hurts a smoker at play. Losing time at work could mean an actual loss in income, depending upon how you are paid. The second table shows that younger smokers are more likely to suffer from a chronic illness and therefore not be able to enjoy the sports or other activities they may like. It means bad news all the way, in your job and for your lifestyle.

Think of it in terms of days you lose from your job or tennis or handball or hiking or whatever else you like to do. Eleven and a half days in bed each year is three weeks in bed every two years. Who needs it, at any age.

So, the facts are that even if cigarette smokers do not die from smoking, they still lose, because they have to spend more time in bed and they are restricted by chronic illness from doing the kinds of things they would like to do.

SUMMARY

On the face of it, the evidence against smoking cigarettes is over-whelming. Not only can cigarettes hurt your ability to enjoy life, whether it is in sports or business or the ability to have children, but they can kill you; and in most unpleasant ways. After all, dying from cancer is not the easiest way to go.

The problem is that people are blindsided by their addiction. I know from my own experience that I wanted a cigarette so badly that I didn't care what the numbers said. And I am a **statistician.** If you smoke, you know what I mean. It is the absolute humiliation of being a slave to a deadly and disgusting habit. I am ashamed to admit it, but I had no way of escape until I found the way described in this book.

I know this method works. If you are careful, and follow my instructions and pay attention to the warnings, you can easily succeed.

How People Start Smoking

N o one is born with a desire to smoke cigarettes. Most people start between the ages of 10 and 20 years. Some of them say that they didn't even enjoy smoking when they started. So why do people start smoking, if they don't like it in the beginning? What gets them started on cigarettes?

The first place I tried to find this out was the Government's Office of Smoking and Health in Maryland. It immediately became apparent that there was little or no data available on teenagers and smoking. There is a good reason for this—the government forbids the companies to study teenage smokers. This creates a much larger gap in the data than one might, at first thought, believe possible.

Why? Because in areas affecting the consumer, commercial research is usually the forerunner and is much more thorough and professional than government or academic research. This is simply because companies watch their markets very closely and must spend the money to get the answers when the subject is important.

Since the cigarette companies are legally forbidden to market to anyone under 21, it means they do not have consumer research on young people. And, incidentally, this is one government restriction the tobacco companies really pay attention to. They never do studies among teenagers, nor do they permit their research suppliers to interview teenagers. If a consumer research supplier accidentally gets **even one** teenager in a sample of 40,000 people being interviewed, the companies order the interview destroyed immediately. They do not want to see it. They do not want to know anything about it. They do not want to know it happened—Even 1 person under 21 in 40,000. The last thing any cigarette manufacturer wants is to be accused of trying to sell teenagers cigarettes.

Anyway, they do not have an absolute need to do the research. Teenager marketing is no secret in the business. The cigarette companies' advertising agencies market other products to teenagers for other clients. The companies themselves have subsidiaries that market to young people. For example, 7 Up was owned by Phillip Morris and Canada Dry is owned by R.J. Reynolds. So, they already know how to appeal to people under twenty-one in their advertising, their promotion and through such things as sponsorship of jazz, rock and country music concerts.

Sports events, such as the Indianapolis 500, tennis challenge competitions, Olympic qualifying matches, and motorcycle races are the kinds of sales promotional efforts particularly sought by tobacco companies because of three factors. The first reason is that they almost always provide a hero competitor, either as a direct or an implied endorser. The second, equally important, consideration is that the companies want the association of their cigarette brands with sports, which are clean, healthy, usually outdoor activities. Since this tends to counteract the negative health aspects of cigarettes by alleviating health concerns, it increases the temptation for young people to smoke. The third reason is that the cigarette companies can (without overtly saying so) endorse sports that tend to attract young people. The brand management people like that. The sooner they can get smokers started on their brand, the longer they will have them as customers.

Because there is so little information available about how and why young people begin smoking, I interviewed about forty-five young people in depth as a way of providing insight into what really gets people to smoke.

There appear to be three major reasons people start smoking cigarettes when they are young—smoking symbolizes adulthood, it is part of the macho image, and it is done in response to peer pressure.

The Desire to be Adult

Adulthood is the great goal of a teenager. And I hurry to add that it is a natural goal—this breaking away from the family unit to become independent, to become self-sufficient, to assert oneself as an individual. There is nothing abnormal or unnatural about the process. It begins gradually and, as the teenager grows older, proceeds in its natural order to ultimately end in the formation of a new family unit.

A very normal part of this process is the gradual shedding of one lifestyle to take up another. By its very nature, this process means that the young person also sheds many of the habits and rules of childhood and takes up those of an adult. As in most growth patterns, there is no set guideline or logic to this progression. Most often the young person goes two steps forward and then one step back. It is an irregular pattern of progression.

Smoking is one of the activities permitted to adults, but not to children. Therefore it becomes, quite naturally, one of the things that young people experiment with as they grow into adulthood. They see it as an "adult" activity. The fact that it has been forbidden for so long makes it almost inevitable that it will be tried. This does not mean that it will be taken up as a habit. In fact, since only about one-third of adults smoke cigarettes, the odds are that the smoking habit will be rejected.

On the other hand, smoking will almost certainly be tried, if only because, like drinking, it symbolizes breaking away, independence, emulating older people, adulthood. This is particularly true if our parents smoke. So the child starts smoking as a way to enter adulthood. It is not a big thing. In the scheme of things, it is only a small symbolic gesture, but to many young people, it is a meaningful gesture.

For example, a young man said in an interview:

> It was part of being a teenager. I smoked. My father offered me $1,000 if I wouldn't smoke until I was 21, but everyone else was smoking. My father smoked. It was a way of growing up, of becoming an adult, and, I guess, of becoming like him. So I did it anyway. I smoked. I couldn't lie to him so I never got the $1,000. I wish I had never started. Now I can't give them up.

A young woman respondent who works as a clerk stated:

I wanted to feel grown-up. It was fun in the beginning. You had a sense of belonging. We were doing what we wanted to do instead of what we were told to do.

A young girl from New Jersey described how she felt at the time in these words:

If an older person wanted to smoke, he could smoke. So why couldn't us kids? It was an older person's rule, that kids couldn't smoke and we weren't kids any more. We were more mature. So we started to act like we were older people; at least, it was our idea of how older people acted. We smoked.

A nineteen-year-old man in the same group stated:

Hell, it was exciting. We were breaking the rules. We were just kids and so—we were doing what adults do. We were trying to be big shots. I remember, I really felt grown up when I reached in my pocket and offered my girl a cigarette.

His wife went on to say:

Oh, it was just part of growing up. Everybody did it. It made us feel older. That's why we did it. Thank God I stopped, but my sister. You should see her. She never stops. The ashtrays in her house are piled with mounds of dead butts—disgusting.

A young man from North Carolina summed it all up in a few words:

My daddy smoked. My granddaddy smoked. My uncle George smoked. I wanted to be like them, so I smoked.

Smoking Is Macho

There is a definite macho symbolism to smoking, and we use the word "macho" in its broadest possible sense—as some sort of a male/female, power/sex symbol. Although no one can prove this empirically, there are strong associative research findings that indicate that the symbolism exists and that it has a dynamic effect upon product and brand purchase.

A strong-tasting cigarette is associated with a strong man and a big cigar is associated with a rich and powerful man, in the same way that the slow-burning pipe is associated with the calm and wise man and a long, thin cigarette is successful only in brands appealing to women. These are physical attributes of a product. However, emotional attributes can be built into a product just as effectively. The cowboy, the sailor, the lumberjack, the white hunter, the motorcyclist and the Eve woman, all of whom are heroes in the cigarette advertisements, are research-proven macho power/sex symbols designed to produce a predisposition toward use on the part of the present or potential smoker.

As one respondent said in an interview:

I smoked because all the guys I knew were doing it. I wanted to be one of them. We would do it in the locker room at school and then we would swagger out—if we didn't get caught that is. It made us feel like big guys, you know, macho.

Later, when shown a Marlboro regular advertisement, he went on to say:

He's a cowboy. He's got a good life, out in the open, riding horses. It's very healthy. What kind of a person is he? I think he's quiet; he looks strong, rugged. Is he tough? Oh yeah, he looks like Clint Eastwood. I wouldn't want to tangle with him on a dark night.

His wife, in the same interview, added:

But I think he would be gentle too. Anyone who is around animals has to be gentle; very protective. I like that.

One man said:

I felt as though I had become somebody the first time I smoked. But you have to remember, I was just a kid. It was a big deal to me then. I felt more like a man. Now it seems stupid.

This man said he started smoking cigarettes because he wanted to look like a man in front of his girl:

My girl, she smoked. She was a year older than me and she was very sophisticated. I wanted to be like her—well, you know, I was going out with her and I didn't want to look like a kid. I wanted to look like I knew what it was all about. So I started smoking with her.

Now here is the other side. A housewife from the North Shore of Long Island talked about how she wanted to show her date that she was right on with the best of them.

> *This guy I was going with: God, was he good-looking. He was into cigarettes and grass. Marijuana terrified me, but I wasn't going to act like a wimp so I smoked a cigarette. It made me feel daring, and it was fun. It was exciting. At first, I didn't inhale, but then I went all the way with the guy. I was smoking like a chimney.*

This woman told how smoking was a part of breaking away from an old-fashioned, conservative family heritage.

> *My family were very old-fashioned and strict with all of us girls. The boys could do pretty much what they wanted—or at least, they could get away with a lot more. It was expected from the boys. But they [my parents] kept a very strict watch on us. We had to be in by a certain hour, long before any of the other members of my class. So when my date offered me a cigarette, it really was, . . . I guess I was being defiant. If my parents had known, we would have gotten it; they would have been so angry.*

When shown a Virginia Slims ad, she smiled and said:

> *That's a lot more truth than you think. It's not the way down here that it is up there where you come from. That's what I smoke and I think that ad is why.*

The macho element is not apparent only in my individual interviews. It also appears in quantitative research when various types of TAT (Thematic Apperception Tests) and other projective tests are used. True, it cannot be definitively proven as a cause and effect. However, many of the studies were conducted clinical designs using appropriate control cells. Because of the associative behavioral and attitudinal data, it is hard to deny that macho symbolism, whether male or female, is inherently one of the factors that encourage consumers to smoke, not only cigarettes, but when properly associated, a particular brand. Thus it is extremely important to marketing and brand management as a sales appeal.

It is no accident that the two most popular cigarettes, Winston and Marlboro, feature virile, masculine men in their advertising. It is a direct appeal to, and association of those brands with, smokers who want a strong macho, power/sex symbolism. Cigarette marketers are not the only ones to use this appeal. Car makers use it too, with their five-on-the-floor stick shift and 0-to-55-mph-in-5-seconds type of advertising.

The power/sex drive is a basic human desire that we all have and that the marketers play to in advertising many, many different kinds of products. It is not confined to men or women. It is universal, appealing equally to both sexes. *Cosmopolitan* uses the theme to perfection on its covers, with a dramatic portrayal of a young independent woman. It is a superb example of the use of the appeal in a product appealing to women. And it works, every month. You know it because *Cosmopolitan* has very few subscription sales. That front cover and the contents have to sell it every single month.

The marketers of cigarettes appealing to women use the female macho sales theme in the same way. Virginia Slims does it with its slogan "You've come a long way, baby," and by showing a strong, virile, attractive woman "doer" in its artwork.

Marlboro uses the theme with strong emphasis on power and a subdued sense of virility and strength as an appeal in its artwork. One of the most interesting things about the Marlboro appeal is that the particular male stereotype—the cowboy is equally appealing to women and to men. On the other hand, this is not true of female models. Research has shown that the use of a female model (cowgirl) in the Marlboro theme attracts only women, and is not very effective even with them.

The images used for Barclay cigarettes perfectly illustrate a more obviously sexual version of the same macho-type appeal. They were chosen brilliantly and deliberately, just as we specified in our recommendations to Brown and Williamson. They use pictures that portray a virile, attractive person in a classically formal, romantic setting with strong sexual overtones and the hint, but not the overt presence, of the opposite sex. Meanwhile the copy concentrates on product attributes, particularly low tar/nicotine and good taste.

Interestingly, in this type of format a female model works just as well attracting women as a male model does in attracting men. There were no apparent differences in the effectiveness of the ads featuring protagonists of each sex, as long as they stuck to the basic theme.

The brand was an instant success.

Peer Pressure

There is no way to underestimate the importance of peer pressure. What the studies indicate is that a young person goes through a thought process that one of them summed up in the following words during one of my interviews. It seems to say it all.

Some of my friends smoked. They were the guys who did everything, who went out with girls. They wanted me to try it. I wanted to be like them—independent, and more like a man. So I did. I took a drag, and after a while I got used to it and I didn't stop.

Another respondent asked him if he had wanted to stop. He went on to describe his friends:

No, not really. These were my friends, and the girl I wanted to date was one of them. There are some guys that are fun and some aren't. These were my kind of guys. Maybe we broke a few rules, but we never hurt anyone. They've all done pretty well, too. One of the guys has a car dealership, another is a big wheel in a New York insurance company. They weren't the kind of guys to sit around and do nothing. I don't mean you had to smoke. It's just that you couldn't be a crump.

Another teenager describes the pressures that friends can put on a nonsmoker when he tells how he started and persisted in smoking even though the first-time trials made him sick.

They [my friends] wanted me to see what it was like. They kept offering me cigarettes. So that's how. I puffed on one. I wanted to be a part of it so I started smoking. It just happened.

In fact, I didn't like cigarettes at all. The first time I tried them, they tasted awful. I was sick to my stomach. I went into the toilet and threw up—and not just once, either. I was really sick. I only started to smoke because I wanted to be one of the guys.

Why did I start? I told you. Everybody else was doing it, so I did it. It was the thing to do. What else?

Also, no one likes to break the rules alone. When you are doing something wrong and you are likely to get punished if you are found out, then it is better to have strength in numbers. At least that way you are not the only one who is going to get caught and punished. You can always use the excuse that there are a lot of others doing the same overstepping of the line. The social nature of beginning to smoke cigarettes shows in this story.

> *It was no fun doing it alone. Because it was forbidden, you had to have it with someone. And I guess there was another reason; it made it more believable; no one could doubt you if there was somebody to back up your story. It was more fun if you had something to share. I think that's it. That's what makes me remember it.*
>
> *We were all down at the beach. There were about twenty of us, counting our dates. We had some beer and it was one of thsoe beautiful summer nights. Nothing rowdy, just fun and horsing around. One of the chicks had a couple of joints and we passed them around. When that was gone everyone went back to smoking cigarettes. That's the first time I ever smoked. Everybody was doing it. It just seemed like natural and I wasn't going to be an oddball—not and be in that group.*

It sounds like a Hollywood movie setting, and he could be talking about how young people get hooked on almost any drug. They could just as well have been starting to snort cocaine, get drunk on alcohol, high on marijuana, sharing heroin or LSD. And that is not far from wrong, because cigarettes contain a drug (nicotine) that addicts people the same way whiskey has a drug (alcohol) that addicts people—except nicotine addicts them much more quickly than alcohol, though nowhere nearly as quickly as cocaine or heroin.

How They Keep You Smoking

L et's face it, the tobacco companies have a problem. They are selling a product that is a poison. It says so right on the box. It says so in every advertisement, in every promotion piece that the companies put out. It has appeared on the evening television news. It has been featured on the front page of every newspaper in the country. Right? Right.

How do they get around it? How do they get people to ignore such a blatant warning? Easy.

Through advertising, promotion, public relations, giveaways and the use of every kind of research and legal aid to help them do everything correctly. They are fantastic.

Basically, since they are very sophisticated marketers, they use their advertising to accomplish two ends. Of course, their primary objective is to get a smoker to buy their brand. But of almost equal importance is their effort to make smoking their brand appear harmless. They take this dual approach because they know that a high proportion of the market is concerned about the negative health aspects of cigarettes. They make a brand appealing to get you to smoke it and they make it look healthy so you don't quit or trade down; and they pinpoint the whole pitch to the particular kind of person that they are out to sell.

When you look at some of the basics about the role of cigarettes in peoples' lives, you see that first of all, they satisfy a person's addiction. After all, that is why an individual smokes. Then the smoker has to pick a certain brand to smoke. Because the marketer wants smokers to pick his brand of cigarette, that is where the fun (or rather the travail) begins for him.

Now, you have to realize that there is not just one market for cigarettes. The market for cigarettes is segmented into what are really a lot of little markets. Why is that true? Because no single brand of cigarettes can appeal to everybody. Different kinds of people simply smoke different brands of cigarettes. Since a brand can not be "all things to all people," it cannot appeal to everybody. For example, a brand cannot be low tar **and** strong tasting. It cannot be sophisticated **and** appeal to blue collar workers. Virginia Slims cigarettes will never appeal to the men who mine coal or build dams and bridges. It has the wrong symbolism, what marketers call the "image." So the marketer has to pick a market segement and try to sell that group of smokers. To do that, he builds the features of his brand—that is the package, the name, the taste, the shape, the advertising—around the kinds of symbolic qualities that will appeal to the group he is trying to sell.

What all of this does is make it harder for you to switch down because, if you have adopted a cowboy (Marlboro) image of yourself, it is difficult to switch to a cityboy sophisticate (Benson & Hedges).

Here are examples of a few image segments:

Outdoor Blue Collar American

Health Concerned

Upper Status Female

Western Macho Romantic

Black American

Upward Mobile Socially/Economically

Macho Modern Female

Bargain Hunters

Modern Intellectual

Symbolically, what are cigarettes? They are a cheap way of telling the world something about yourself. Every time a smoker takes a package out of his pocket, he is telling the world, this is an image of who I am (or would like to be).

In a way, a package of cigarettes is like a personal status button, except that you don't wear the package on your lapel, you carry it in your pocket and use it to satisfy your addiction. You can display the button whenever you want to by offering someone a smoke.

The president's secretary smokes a Parliament or an Eve. The health-concerned person smokes a Carlton or a Now. The outdoor, blue-collar American smokes a Winston. The All American Western Macho Romantic smokes a Marlboro. The black American smokes a Kool. The up-and-coming young executive smokes a Merit or a Vantage. The chief legal counsel smokes a pipe and the chairman of the board smokes a big, long black cigar. They are all smoking what they think is their image.

So, there is a strong sense of personal image that runs throughout the whole panoply of cigarette brands and types of smoking habits. A large part of this image has to do with its reflections of one's status, be it social status, or peer group, business, money/power, intellectual or some other type of status.

Here are some of the associations that people make to the names of the leading brands.

NAME ASSOCIATION

Brand	Association	Type of Status
Marlboro	Duke of Marlboro	Power/Social Status
Winston	Sir Winston Churchill	Power/Hero
Salem	All American	American Peer Group
Kent	Dukes of Kent	Social Status
Parliament	English Status	Social Status
Merit	Upward Mobile	Achiever/Doer
Carlton	Fancy English Name	Social Status
Now	Modernity	Intellectual
Newport	Rich Man's Resort	Social
Kool	Black Idiom	Black Peer Group
Yves' Ritz	High Style	Stylish Upper Class

Bearing in mind that cigarettes really are slow poisons, these brand names do not sound like poisons. In fact, they all sound and are quite safe and respectable. For the most part, they are all good, solid, high-status, Anglo/Saxon names. You probably think that the names are chosen by accident, or just because they have a nice sound to them. Not so; names may have been chosen that way in years past, but to my knowledge, names have not been chosen that way by big companies for many, many years. Today they are sometimes computer-generated, but from wherever they evolve they are subjected to intensive consumer research involving every aspect of the image they transmit to the smokers they seek to attract.

Once a name is chosen it can't very well be changed, so Name Studies are a very big thing in market research and with management. My husband ran the first study Esso did when they changed their name to Exxon but an executive at the company told him they had over 20 studies in total made before they finally changed their name.

When the management of one company was looking for a new name for one of their cigarettes, we did the first basic study. Then they had some additional questions, so we did the study over again, with a slightly different twist. Then, wanting just to confirm our work, they commissioned another company to design a third study, using a totally different technique, to double check the work we had done.

They were very open about it. "Don't take offense," they said. "We are just being careful to make sure we are right. We always do this. It is no reflection on you."

That's not what we thought. We thought they didn't believe us and were trying to find fault with our work. We looked on the other research company with all the joy of a victim watching a Mafia hit man. We felt a little better when we found out that it really was standard practice and that they were not really trying to find fault with what we had done. (The additional work confirmed our findings).

Advertising

Now, let's look at the advertising themes companies use to sell some of the brands. For reasons not hard to imagine, you will find that almost all of them suggest something healthy, clean, pure, athletic, virile, strong and totally uncorrupted. Because of the need to counteract the poison declarations of the government, the American Cancer Society and the Heart and Emphysema Associations, they sell health, health and more health, usually in conjunction with the great outdoors.

It is a hard sell. By that I mean that the cigarette companies bang it home in their ads. Every cigarette manufacturer does it, and, for the most part, they do it brilliantly. There is no conspiracy because it is simply not a secret in the industry that this kind of campaign works. It works because it overcomes people's fears about smoking and makes all the opposing claims about the dangers of cigarettes seem irrational and overdone.

The Marlboro Man

This is probably the most famous campaign in contemporary cigarette advertising. It took Marlboro from a woman's cigarette (it used to be sold with a red tip to match women's lipstick) to a full-fledged All-American product that is the largest selling brand of cigarettes in the U.S. today.

What do they sell? They sell the cowboy. The American version of the white knight of the fairy tales. They sell by associating the cigarette with a symbol of strength, virility, health and athletic prowess. The All-American symbol of the All-American hero.

Macho? Indeed he is macho. Who could imagine the American cowboy as a wimp?

Now how could the American cowboy be associated with poisons? To say so would be to deny the American Ideal. He is the exact opposite of poisonous. He is wholesome and pure. He is the Sir Gawain of American folklore, and like Sir Gawain, he loves only his horse. You never see a woman in a Marlboro advertisement. Not a temptation to be seen anywhere.

Not only that, but look at the setting. What could be healthier than the great plains and mountain valleys of our American West, with all the fresh, clean air and sunshine and not a speck of smog from factories or automobile exhausts to pollute the atmosphere, just a faint wisp of smoke from a Marlboro.

How could one thin wisp of smoke from a Marlboro cigarette possibly harm anyone in that kind of a setting. Of course, no one could believe that it will. No one looking at the advertisement would ever think that smoking a Marlboro is anything else but the most normal, harmless, healthy thing for an idealistic, hero-worshipping American male to relax in doing. Looking at the ad, how could anyone think otherwise. It is a great sales theme and it is brilliantly executed. The campaign is just marvelous.

Not only that, but if you are the least bit concerned that Marlboros are too strong for you, they have a complementary campaign for Marlboro Lights.

All right, you tell me. What do you think that they do for Marlboro Lights? Well, they minimize the emphasis given to the symbol of strength in the ad (the cowboy) and they emphasize the great Western outdoors using magnificent, four-color, double-page spreads. While this keeps the Western association with Marlboro, it also portrays Marlboro Lights as more strongly associated with the pure, absolutely clean air, open plains and unsullied mountains of the West. And best of all, just to top it off, they usually add a herd of wild horses to emphasize freedom from care.

What could be possibly wrong with smoking a Marlboro Light in that setting—or imagining that setting—every time a person smokes a Marlboro Light. Does this sound poisonous? Of course not. It is beautiful. It is perfect. As a great extension of a marvelous selling theme, it works in the marketplace like an absolute charm, making Marlboro Lights the largest selling brand in its tar/nicotine category in the country.

And at Phillip Morris they know it. To protect their franchise they test almost every ad and every change, because they know that as long as cowboys are American heroes, they have a winner. All they have to do is keep it rolling and not make any mistakes. So they are very thorough in their consumer-advertising research. Cost is not a problem. They just need to make sure they have the very best.

For now, let us look at just a few more of the advertising campaigns cigarette companies have designed for their brands. In reading my New York *Daily News*, I come to a full-page black-and-white advertisement for Parliament Lights. The advertisement shows a man and a woman relaxing on the beach of a very small tropical island. The palm trees are blowing in the wind and the cumulus clouds in the background are scudding across a bright, clear tropical sky.

Here again we have a "clear air" theme, except that it uses a tropical island instad of the Great American West to portray the idea that smoking is not incompatible with health. We see lots of fresh air, sunshine, tropical breezes, clean untouched white beaches on a

sparkling ocean, a relaxed, carefree young couple in bathing suits—
in short, all of the ingredients that are needed to allay any smokers'
fears that might be aroused by the mandatory government warning
at the bottom of the page:

*SURGEON GENERAL'S WARNING: Smoking Causes Lung Cancer,
Heart Disease, Emphysema, And May Complicate Pregnancy.*

Why, a wisp of cigarette smoke wouldn't last a second in all
those ocean breezes. Who could imagine cigarettes, even a pack or
a carton, being dangerous in a setting like that?

And to reinforce the impact of the pictorial message, the copy
goes on to imply the effectiveness of the patented Parliament filter.
It reads, "A unique filter for extra smooth taste and low tar enjoyment." Now what could be more harmless than that? Low tar too.
My, my.

Now, you are probably laughing at me for writing all of this and
thinking to yourself that I am exaggerating—or that I am being
sarcastic or facetious. But the very real truth of the matter is that it
works. In the real world, it sells cigarettes—a high-status name; a
good-tasting, low-tar cigarette with a special filter; a clean healthy
image symbolized by a tropical island and an attractive person of
the opposite sex in a bathing suit with whom to enjoy it all. That's
the message in the ad ... and it works. For the people who want
that imagery, it sells cigarettes. People take money out of their purse
and pocket, and they put it down on the counter to pay for
Parliament Light cigarettes. That is the bottom line. After all, how
could anyone associate lung cancer with a product like the Parliament Lights cigarettes as portrayed in the ad.

Let us take a quick look at the Merit appeal since it is quite close
to the Parliament Lights' pitch. Merit cigarettes use action photos
of sailboats in the open ocean. They are big sailboats manned by
handsome young men who can presumably afford them. They
portray the active life of the rich, successful, up-and-coming executive. There you have an ocean theme like the Parliament Lights
advertisement, with all the same connotations of clean living but
aimed at the up-and-coming action people rather than the con-
tented people who sit on the beach and "have it made." But the
same emphasis on wholesomeness is there, deliberately designed to
counter the negative health implications of cigarettes.

At the far, low end of the market is what the industry has

dubbed the "Health Concerned Smoker." While these people want to smoke and they haven't decided how to quit, they are the group that is most afraid of getting cancer or some other dread disease. The cigarette companies appeal to these health concerned smokers with a pseudo-scientific series of advertisements describing how much lower in tar they are (and presumably better for your health). For example, the Carlton slogan is "If You Smoke, Please Try Carlton."

But at the same time, Carlton and Now both do their very best to fool you. They will bang the poor smokers up from a .1 to .6 mg nicotine habit every chance they get, and the smokers will fall for it almost every time unless they know what you learned from reading about tricks and traps earlier in the book.

Do Smokers Believe Smoking Is Harmful?

S o why do we smoke? When we know that the results are so dreadful. Don't we believe all those years of testing among millions of people? Don't they often see the cancer epidemic among their friends with their own eyes?

There is no data available, at least that I could find, describing whether smokers "believe" cigarettes are harmful. The government does not appear to have done any research on the subject. I have been told by the research people at the tobacco companies that they all regularly research the problem. However, anything to do with health is a sensitive subject, and all studies of this type are conducted using a technique called "focused group interviews." The reports are submitted orally and no records are ever kept of this kind of sensitive work, lest they be subpoenaed by the government or people suing the cigarette companies.

Therefore this chapter is based on my own interviews. These were exploratory and designed to determine how people felt rather than try to take a measure of the entire country. To obtain the material I conducted six focused group interviews and fifteen depth interviews among cigarette smokers, using non-directed techniques.

What this means is that I interviewed people in a group and encouraged them to talk informally about what they believed or did not believe and why, without asking a lot of specific questions. In this way, we learn what **they** want to talk about rather than what we think is important. A total of seventy-one smokers were interviewed in the focused groups. In order to get a variety of opinions, I deliberately chose smokers of cigarettes with different tar/nicotine levels from a variety of social and economic backgrounds so that I could have as much input as possible.

What emerges from the group interviews is that almost all smokers we interviewed believe that cigarette smoking is bad for their health. Actually, studies by the American Cancer Society show that 90% of smokers have tried to quit but failed to do so. On the other hand, it is also true that a small minority of smokers are unconcerned and have no interest in quitting. The intensity of smokers' opinions is not a clear-cut, black-and-white set of opinions, but one made up of an infinite series of grays.

Most of the cigarette smokers we interviewed were afraid of smoking. They fear for their health, but they do not actually know how much of a risk it is to smoke cigarettes. Many people were confused by the ambiguous role of the government. On one hand, the government condemns smoking; on the other hand, it does nothing to prevent it, and in fact actively subsidizes the growing and the price of tobacco. Many smokers seemed to believe that smoking was not really "that" bad for your health. If it were, the government would "do something" about preventing it. As one respondent put it: "If they did all that research and they know it is bad for people, why don't they ban it?" It is also noteworthy that richer people and particularly better-educated, up-and-coming young people seemed to be more conscious of the health dangers and more intent on quitting smoking.

A young, upwardly mobile junior executive said:

I believe the studies. I know I shouldn't smoke, but I like it. I tried to quit last fall, but it was no good. We were doing an important merger then and the pressure at the office was just fierce. I was working seven days a week. I mean Sundays too. It was just the wrong time. Yes, I am going to give it up. It's not healthy and I know it and doesn't do my jogging any good, but I've got to find a time when things quiet down.

A long-time smoker who is a statistical consultant said:

They (cigarettes) are dangerous. I should start to leave off, but I never do it.

You read a lot of stories on smoking. You know people die sooner, but you don't believe it will happen to me. Here I am in the statistical consulting business, and emotionally, I don't believe it will ever happen to me. Now isn't that stupid?

A young mother in one of the interviews, said:

I know, I know. The doctor told me I should stop when I got pregnant again. He said that it wasn't good for the baby, but we're moving to the new house. I don't think it's going to hurt the baby that much. Mother smoked when she had us. We're fine.

I don't understand the pamphlets (my doctor gave me) anyway. I read all of them in his office, but I don't understand them. Anyway, isn't it better if the baby doesn't weigh as much? I like to smoke, especially when my husband is away travelling."

Interestingly, we found considerable peer pressure to stop smoking. While it seems most evident among young, up-and-coming white-collar smokers, it is present among all groups. Here are some of the comments by the smokers who attended the group sessions.

It has gotten so that almost none of my friends smoke. I'm one of the few. You go to a party and almost nobody smokes. I had a girl tell me that she couldn't live with a smoker. She said it was a dirty habit.

A nonsmoking IBM salesman said:

If you are on the [tennis] courts all day, very few people smoke. It's bad for your wind, especially if you are playing singles. Look at the people here, just talking or waiting for a court. How many do you see smoking? We frown on that. It sets a bad example for the young people.

A lower-income black man who works in a garage says:

My wife won't leave me alone about it and my kids tell me how bad it is, but I need it. They all say it's not good for my coughin', but I cain't not do it. I know they are right but do it anyway.

People who believe the data become more concerned about their health. These people tend to choose a "healthier" cigarette. This is extremely important to cigarette companies because it affects the brands of cigarettes people smoke. Research has proven that the more smokers are concerned about the effects of smoking on their health, the more likely they are to use low-tar cigarettes, like Carlton or Now. The less concerned they are about the effects of smoking on their health, the more likely they are to smoke a strong cigarette like a Marlboro or a Winston.

Smokers who are more health concerned are already switching down to brands with lower tar/nicotine levels. As one woman who lived in an upper-income New York suburb said:

> Frightened, I'm scared to death. My mother and my grandmother both died of cancer. It scares me. I have got to quit.
>
> Why? I'm afraid of it. It was awful what they went through. It scares me. I will [quit] one of these days. I smoke Benson & Hedges Ultra Lights now. I'm trying to give them up.

A salesman stated:

> I love smoking. I like the taste. I like the feeling of smoking. I've been smoking since I was a young kid—but now I'm afraid of them. You read all the stories about cancer and it starts to frighten you. My grandmother used to call cigarettes 'coffin nails.' Maybe they are just beginning to prove she was right. I worry sometimes.

On the other hand, blue-collar workers and those who were less well educated did not seem to think that smoking was as dangerous as did white-collar workers—or that the need to quit was as great. To some extent, this may be a matter of literacy and reading interests.

Also, I have found in the course of my work that it is difficult for many people to understand abstract statistical figures and the way they can have a real-life impact on one's business, one's health, and one's investments. For example, I have a friend who was left a lot of money twenty years ago and has kept it all in CDs and money market funds. These were very safe investments, but she spent only the interest she got from them. So she still has the same amount of money, but because of inflation it buys only 40 percent of what it used to. She has had to go back to work. She can't understand the consequences of statistics: that a 6 percent inflation rate means that her money loses 45 percent of its purchasing power every ten years. It can be hard to grasp reality in the form of funny little percentages.

In addition, it is my personal opinion that their addiction prevents many smokers from seeing reality. Many, many smokers must know that smoking cigarettes is harmful to their health. They have been warned, but I think their addiction keeps them from the truth; that they keep telling themselves, as one respondent (a surgeon) in an interview says: "Maybe it is statistically true, but that doesn't mean it will happen to me."

Part of the problem is statistics, because statistics are hard to relate to. But there is a large element of self-delusion here as well. Read the following conversation by some women smokers in New Jersey after they are shown some of the figures in the Surgeon General's report. The first woman laughed nervously and said:

> I don't want to believe it. If smoking is that dangerous, I'd have to give it up.

Then she begins to rationalize and said:

> If it is that dangerous the government wouldn't allow it. Why doesn't the government stop it? I don't think it is that dangerous.

Another woman, in the same interview, broke in:

> But those are government figures. They come from the Government.

The first woman answered back, ducking the whole issue:

> Well, I don't care. People can play all kinds of games with numbers. I still say, if it's that bad the Government wouldn't let people smoke. It would pass a law against cigarettes.

In another interview, a construction worker said:

> No one has ever proved smoking causes cancer. Even the government can't prove it and they spent millions of dollars. I don't believe that anyone knows what causes cancer. Prove it and I will stop smoking. Until they prove it, I'm going to smoke all I want.
>
> I'm not finished yet. The whole thing is unconstitutional. I have to sit in a separate section in the theater, or on a bus. Now they want me to sit in another part of the restaurant. I object to that. No one has proved what makes cancer.

Another respondent asked, "How about radiation. That causes cancer?"

> I suppose you are going to tell me cigarettes make radiation. I like to

smoke and I'm going to smoke. That's my business. You mind your business and I'll mind mine.

If they find one claim about the health dangers of smoking unbelievable, some confirmed smokers will reject all the good arguments put forth so that they can continue with their habit. This kind of thinking shows in this quotation:

Some doctor in California says that if you are in the same room with someone smoking, you'll get cancer. Do you believe that? I don't. When you try and pin them down, none of these anti-smoking nuts have any proof.
    If smoking is that bad, the government would stop selling cigarettes.

Other people are just plain fatalistic about the effects of smoking and don't seem to believe that it will matter one way or another:

I like smoking. I'm not in the mind to quit. What difference does it make? I'm going to die of something anyway. I'd rather live my life the way I like. I don't believe all that Ralph Nader stuff anyway. Life is too short to worry about all that talk.

A man who lives in Lancaster, Pennsylvania, said:

I own some stock in R.J. Reynolds. I read in the Annual Report that the president said that if somebody would tell him what chemicals in cigarettes cause cancer he will take them out of all R.J. Reynolds cigarettes immediately. No one has told him anything [in cigarettes] causes cancer.

Young people in particular don't seem to want to worry about the health effects of cigarettes. One father got this from his nineteen-year-old daughter when he spoke to her about the dangers of smoking: "Oh, Daddy, nobody ever thinks about things like that."

A teenage respondent said:

Cancer? Aah, that's for old people. Who gets cancer when they are my age? Nobody. I'll quit when I get old, around forty, maybe.

Another young person stated:

Smoking hurts my handball? Who said so? Nobody told me. The government warnings? I never read them. I never read that stuff. What they say. If I smoke a cigarette, I'm going to die. I don't believe it.

A young mother said:

I know it's not good for me, but right now, I'm too busy. I've got three children to take care of and we're trying to get the farmstand going. It's too much to think about. I'm not going to die of cigarettes, not this year, anyway.

So it is the old story. No one wants to face bad news until it is too late.

But it is more than that too. Because people **are** confused. The government, to whom everyone looks as the great and all-knowing father, is ambiguous in dealing with the cigarette-smoking problem. The Agriculture Department subsidizes tobacco and the Surgeon General, who guards the nation's health, decries the use of the product from every pulpit he can find.

Television is not allowed to accept cigarette advertising, but we see a double-page, four-color Marlboro spread almost every time we open a magazine. Even worse, if we read the editorial on the page next to the Marlboro ad, there is probably an article by a doctor pointing out the dangers of even sitting next to someone who is smoking.

This has its effects. As Pavlov teaches us, alternating approval and disapproval (punishment) signals confuse people and render them incapable of making decisions. Obviously people can still make rational decisions about their health, but the confusing signals emanating from the government and the media do tend to create doubts in people's minds about the dangers of smoking.

No one, even the most fanatical anti-smoking crusader, wants the atmosphere that total prohibition would bring, but still there is room for the government to take a sensible and united stand against a major health hazard. That is going to be difficult for the government. The Tobacco Senators will rally stridently against any limitations on cigarette advertising or tobacco subsidies. Smoking brings in millions of dollars in taxes and the tobacco companies' profits finance literally hundreds of political campaigns. The problem is that money and power speak loudly, even when it is the nation's health at stake.

CHAPTER ELEVEN

Profits & Politics

W hy does America permit the open, advertised sale of a product with such horrible consequences. There are a number of reasons: the importance of the tobacco crop and the tobacco industry and the taxes they bring to federal, state and local governments. But one of the most important is—money.

The profits of the tobacco companies are almost beyond belief. Anyone who becomes involved in cigarette marketing is immediately stunned by the enormity of profits in the business. These profits are so great that they boggle the mind, even for someone like myself, who has spent my working life in consumer package goods marketing.

It is these huge profits that make the tobacco companies almost invulnerable to attack, that enable them to spend enormous sums for lobbying against anti-cigarette laws, for legal services to protect themselves against lawsuits, for advertising and promotion to protect and maintain their share of the market, for the free giveaway packages that they hand out on the street to get you to try their brand and, most important of all, for political contributions.

There is no secret about the profit picture, it is all in their annual reports. We will give you examples from two of their annual reports later in this chapter. However, since it is always easier for me to think in terms of my own pocketbook, let me first try to explain the profitability of cigarettes starting from the point of view of the individual smoker's pocketbook.

Think of it this way. As of July 1986 a cigarette company sells its brands for an average of $34.72 per 1,000 or 61 cents a pack net to the company after federal excise taxes. If you smoke a pack a day, or 365 packs a year, that is $222.65 income for the cigarette company. Now, obviously all of that is not profit. But their profit from you, just one smoker, is about $100.00 per year, per smoker—and there are conservatively 50 million smokers!

What that means is that 1 percent of market, or 500,000 smokers, is worth a profit in the neighborhood of $50 million a year; profit—not gross—net bottom-line profit, depending on how efficient an operation the company runs.

To a cigarette brand manager, this means that if he or she increases the brand's share of market by just 1 percent of market (1 share point, as they say in the industry), his company makes about an additional $50 million profit. Do you wonder that the brand managers watch their advertising and sales with such microscopic care? If a brand manager comes up with a good idea, or one that even looks good, the companies will give him all the money he or she needs to test it, and a nice fat bonus if it works.

The 1984 report of the error Federal Trade Commission states that Brown and Williamson spent $150 million to introduce Barclay cigarettes. Now I really don't think they spent that much. Not including test marketing, my own guess would be that they spent around $60 or $75 million, but no more than that. The difference between my estimates and the FTC estimates is probably that I think they target marketed, whereas the FTC would have assumed they went totally national.

But even assuming the FTC is right, all they needed to do was pick up 2 percent of market and they would have had their whole $150 million investment in the Barclay introduction back in eighteen months—one and a half years—from just 2 percent of market! Do you believe it? Incredible.

That is how profitable it is to be in the tobacco business.

That is why they have the money to spend.

That is why they are so tough to beat, legally, in the marketplace, politically, at public relations, or any other way.

That is also why the cigarette companies are so incredibly careful about everything they do and why they spend so much on consumer surveys. The fact of that kind of money at stake when the dice are rolled also tells you why the marketing management is the best that money can buy. You probably thought I was over-emphasizing when I wrote about their professionalism. But I was not. The staffs are very good and they are fun to work with because they are very good. It is always much nicer to work with pros than with amateurs. They are a joy because they know their business so well. It is like watching the smooth grace of an Arnold Palmer as he puts the ball on the pin every time. He makes it look so easy. There is never any discussion of what club to use or how to play the shot because he knows exactly what has to be done and how to do it.

There is another reason the companies keep making more money even though total consumption is flat. They keep raising the price on the smoker. Since over 40 percent of the price is sales taxes, only about half the price increase hits the smoker in his pocketbook.

A brand research manager had this in mind when she pointed out to me one day that despite all the published bad news, it hadn't stopped people from smoking. Her firm was making more money than ever, and she said that they raised the price every time they could, never too much at once, just a little bit at a time. But since they were selling to people who are addicted, they'd continue to smoke unless the company hit them with too much of a price increase at one time.

Now, we shall take a look at the corporate reports of the two largest cigarette companies, Phillip Morris, the company that owns Marlboro, Merit, and Benson & Hedges; and R.J. Reynolds, the company that owns Winston, Salem, Vantage, and Now, to see just how much money each company is making.

In their 1985 annual report, Phillip Morris states that "Market share for Phillip Morris U.S.A. rose .06 share points in 1985 to approximately 35.9 percent. ... Operating income for 1985 climbed 17.5 percent to $2.1 billion." In other words, Phillip Morris made an operating profit of $58.5 million dollars for every 1 percent of market.

R.J. Reynolds, in their 1985 annual report, stated that their market share was 31.6% and their operating income was $1.5 billion. This works out to a profit of $47.5 million dollars for every 1 percent of market. This means that just these two companies made over $3.6 billion profit in 1985, over 95 percent of which came from cigarettes. The figures for the two companies are compared here:

CIGARETTE COMPANY EARNINGS

Company	Earnings ($ Billions)	Market Share (per cent)	Earnings Per Share Point ($ Millions)
Phillip Morris	2.1	35.9	58.5
R.J. Reynolds	1.5	31.6	47.5
Total	3.6	67.5	NA

Source: 10K Reports to the Securities and Exchange Commission (SEC)

Operating revenues for Phillip Morris U.S.A. in 1985 rose 7.8 percent while operating income rose 17.5 percent. R.J. Reynolds (U.S.A.) fared similarly to Phillip Morris in 1985. To quote their annual report "Earnings from operations rose 13 percent on sales that were 3.7 percent higher." Earnings for both companies rose more than twice as fast as sales.

Where does the money go? Some of it goes to the shareholders in dividends. A lot of it goes to buy other companies. Phillip Morris owns Miller Brewing and 7 Up. It just bought General Foods for $5.6 billion, which means that it has added Post Cereals, Maxwell House, Jello, Birdseye, Entenmanns, Oscar Mayer, Sanka and over 50 other brands to its roster of products.

For its part, R.J. Reynolds owns Del Monte, Sunkist, Grey Poupon, Hawaiian Punch, Canada Dry, Kentucky Fried Chicken and A1 Sauce. It just bought Nabisco for $2.5 billion, which includes Planters Peanuts, Blue Bonnet and Fleischmann Margarines, Oh Henry and the whole Fleischmann Liquor division, to add to Heublein Liquors it already owns.

Where does the money come from and why did profits go up so much faster than sales? Well, it comes from your pockets, and, of course, both companies raised their cigarette prices substantially in 1985. We suppose that if you are going to spend $5.6 billion to buy General Foods or $2.5 billion to buy Nabisco, you have to raise the price a little. R.J. Reynolds' report to the Securities and Exchange Commission states that they spent $500 million and borrowed $2.0 billion to buy Nabisco. (Remember what that research brand manager said about being able to raise the price when you needed a little extra money, for example, to buy General Foods or Nabisco.) Smokers, they have you hooked.

You pay them very well for your addiction to smoking their brands. They pick your pockets even better.

PROFITS AND POLITICS

Every time there is an anti-tobacco proposal, a cigarette tax hike proposed, or any law to restrict smoking, cries of the wounded tobacco politicians echo throughout the land agonizing over the terrible restrictions on personal liberty or the dreadful, unfair taxes that are imposed on the tobacco farmer.

These men are so powerful (Jesse Helms is the ranking Republican member of the Senate Agriculture Committee and Strom Thurmond is head of the Senate Judiciary Committee) that they not only succeeded in getting the tobacco subsidies increased but also almost managed to get the federal tax on cigarettes cut in half. They did all this at a time when budget deficits were going to over $200 billion a year.

Why is the tobacco lobby so powerful?

Tobacco begins with the U.S. farmer, who is already beset with grievous economic woes because of the collapse of grain and meat prices. Tobacco employs over 100,000 farmers full time and, according to the Wharton School, provides another 400,000 people with part-time jobs during the tobacco harvest and curing season. It is the main prop to the farm economy in North and South Carolina, Kentucky, Tennessee and Virginia. It is also grown in seventeen other states and as far south as Puerto Rico and as far north as Hartford, Connecticut. In 1983 the tobacco harvest generated over $2.4 billion of farm income, $1 billion for North Carolina farmers alone. Kentucky's share that year was $800 million, according to the U.S. Department of Agriculture.

Growing tobacco is hard work. It takes a lot of hand labor to harvest, about 250 hours per acre, according to the Tobacco Institute. This makes it ideal for small farmers, because the post-harvesting preparation and curing can be done by family members or by using part-time labor.

If it takes all that work, why do farmers continue to grow tobacco? Easy. Tobacco is very profitable, and the more of the hand labor a farmer or his family can do on their own, the more profitable it becomes. Tobacco today, like corn whiskey in colonial times, pays the largest part of the farmer's bills. For example, corn sells for about $3.30 per bushel or, at 100 bushels to the acre, an income of $330 per acre. On the other hand, tobacco sells for $1.95 a pound and at 2,000 pounds per acre has an income of $3900 per acre.

The average flue-cured tobacco farm only has about 16 acres, mainly because of the government's policy of strict acreage allotments. By contrast, the average wheat farm is over 300 acres, and wheat takes only about 3 hours per acre to harvest. Tobacco is so profitable you need a government permit to grow it, and there are very strict and severe penalties for overplanting.

Which would you grow on a small farm with a limited allotment: corn at $330 income per acre or tobacco at $3,900 per acre? Need I ask?

If you have the government permit to grow tobacco, just renting out your tobacco land to tenant farmers will bring better than $1,750 per acre. On an average 16-acre tobacco farm that will bring you $28,000 per year without lifting a finger. So if you can get a bunch of government permits to grow tobacco, you can make a nice living just renting out the land to tenants. Without the price supports and the acreage limitations, the tobacco farm economy would be forced to go to larger farms and mechanize production and the price of tobacco would drop rapidly.

Since agriculture is only one small part of the picture, here is a table showing the impact of tobacco on the economy as a whole.

IMPACT OF TOBACCO ON THE NATIONAL ECONOMY

Business	People Employed	Wages Paid ($ Billions)	Sales Value ($ Billions)
Agriculture	100,000	.701*	2.4**
Manufacturing	76,900	2.837	8.6
Federal Excise Tax	NA	NA	4.8
Wholesale Trade	35,357	.884	4.0
State Excise Tax	NA	NA	4.2
Retail Trade	192,720	2.303	3.4
Retail Sales Tax	NA	NA	.8
Total	414,217	$6.726	$28.2
Less Excise and Sales Taxes			-$ 9.8
Net Direct Contribution			$18.4

*Total wages from agriculture and auctions.
**Auction value
NA: Not Applicable.
Source: Chase Econometrics Study for the Tobacco Institute, Database 1983

Taxes

What the preceding table shows is that excise and sales taxes take the largest portion of the smoker's cigarette dollar, $9.8 billion, or 35 percent. The reason we separated out these taxes is that they are, in effect, a hidden sales tax of almost $10 billion that smokers are subjected to every time they buy a pack or a carton of cigarettes. Incidentally, excise taxes are not income taxes and they are not paid by the companies. They are paid by the smokers. The companies merely collect the taxes for the government and pass the cost along to the smoker. This is a sizable contribution to federal, state and local governments, and the tobacco industry's role as a hidden tax collector is a big reason why politicians do not crack down harder on the industry.

Manufacturing and Farming

When the hidden sales taxes are subtracted out, the tobacco industry's contribution to the economy is $18.4 billion. Manufacturing takes the biggest portion of this money, $8.6 billion, or 47 percent. The farmer gets $2.4 billion, or 13 percent. This is only about a quarter of the slice that manufacturers get from the tobacco pie.

It should also be said that tobacco products and their attendant services are a major source of foreign trade earnings by the United States and are a considerable aid in reducing the foreign trade deficit. In 1985, 31 percent of the United States tobacco crop was exported. Total exports of tobacco goods and services amounted to $2.7 billion. The United States also imported $0.6 billion during the same year, leaving a net foreign trade surplus for tobacco of $2.1 billion, thus reducing our foreign trade deficit by that amount during the year. This has a dark side, however; the tobacco people argue that it is hypocritical for us to discourage the use of tobacco products to protect our own citizens at home, while we encourage the purchase of our tobacco products abroad in order to increase our exports.

Employment

Looking at another aspect of the Chase study, we find that the tobacco industry accounts for the employment of approximately

414,000 people, or about one person out of 200, or .46 percent of people employed nationally, depending on which way you want to look at it. Interestingly, despite the high wages paid to executives, the tobacco industry accounts for only .34 percent of total wages. This reflects the high proportion of low-paid service workers in the industry, and means that except for the big salaries of the executives and the marketing and advertising people, the average tobacco worker is less well paid than the average American.

Wages

The Chase study shows that tobacco generates $6.7 billion in wages to workers. As would be expected, the manufacturing sector of the tobacco business was responsible for the largest amount of wages paid, $2.8 billion. Retail trade was a close second at $2.3 billion, wholesale trade was third with $0.9 billion and the least wages were paid by farmers, $0.7 billion. This points up the high use of family help that is said to be used by small farmers raising tobacco.

Although it is impossible for me to make exact direct comparisons because we don't have all the data, I did find that manufacturing profits are about $5.0 billion, out of net sales of about $11 billion, so that it appears the industry has a very high profit margin indeed.

All of this gives the industry considerable political clout, and the clout is managed by the cigarette manufacturers and their lobbyists, the Tobacco Institute, because they are the largest organized sector of the industry. A brand manager told me one day after the office had closed and we were chewing the fat, smoking up a storm, trying out a couple of new blends they had going out for product testing, that they had pulled out every political stop they had in 1985, when there was a movement afoot to put cigarettes under the FDA (Food and Drug Administration). This would have meant that all ingredients and the tar and nicotine strength would have to be listed on each package, as is required for food, plus extensive testing and approvals. With cigarettes under the FTC, as they are now, they don't have to list anything. And our colleague was hopeful that political pressure, applied without too much publicity, would get the FTC testing stopped. It appears that they've been at least partly effective, since the FTC has taken a new stance in refusing to release the information on testing.

Of course, the cigarette companies have sound competitive reasons for not wanting to list their ingredients on the package, especially for brands in the Ultra Low segment of the market that uses the highest proportion of taste enhancers and tobacco substitutes. If a cigarette company does discover a uniquely desirable taste appeal, they certainly do not want to broadcast it to their competitors in the industry. Neither would they want to list the chemicals and taste enhancers they use the same way that the food companies have to list chemical additives, even if they are only added to the packaging.

But overall the tobacco companies are in a very favorable position in regard to government regulations. Despite the fact that smokers inhale the smoke into their bodies and despite all the negative publicity, they have been able to maintain their favored position as one of the most unregulated (but highly taxed) consumer products industries in America.

CHAPTER TWELVE

The Battle Joined – The Next Steps

There are two giants locked in conflict. On one side, it is a struggle for people's health; on the other, for their pocketbooks.

The health establishment is pitted against the tobacco industry. For the tobacco industry, it is a bitter battle for survival. Jobs are at stake here, a paycheck and a livelihood. And people will fight savagely to protect these things because their homes, their families, the education of their children, the very blood and marrow of their lives are all at risk.

The people of the tobacco industry are doing just that. They have enormous power through the wealth they extract from the addicts they supply. The roles played by entrenched political interests persuading the FTC to stop publishing the levels of tar and nicotine in cigarettes is just one example of their effectiveness.

If you question the importance of having the FTC continue to publish tar/nicotine levels, let me point out one fact: Since the FTC has stopped publishing the tar/nicotine data, **10 out of 12 of the tar/nicotine changes I could identify have been up. Almost every brand that changed has increased its addiction level.**

The most powerful force harrying the tobacco industry and their political minions is the health establishment, primarily the American Medical Society, the American Cancer Society and the

American Lung Association. They may have enormous public support but they do not have the power or the money of the tobacco
groups—nor of addicts whose pockets they can pick for a daily
income.

These organizations are active defenders of the public interest.
For the most part, they act wihout hope of private gain. Many are
paid nothing. There are few rewards for what they do. The nameless
doctors and administrators who lead this fight will not receive so
much as a scrap of paper to hang on their walls; Ronald Reagan
gives no Freedom Medals to people who attack the tobacco industry.
They are the real heroes who give, as it says in the Talmud, without
hope even of recognition. If they can stop these merchants of
disease, they will save more lives than Jonas Salk with less credit
than I will get for this small paperback book.

Public safety is the issue here—not the addiction of the individual smoker or the danger he does to his person. Only when
public safety is endangered do cigarettes become a matter of public
policy. This is true of smoking, just as it is true for alcohol. During
Prohibition this country went through the trauma of a crusade in
the attempt ot prevent people from harming themselves by drinking; it was a terrible failure. It is doubtful that we will ever make
the same mistake again and unilaterally forbid the use of cigarettes.
But that does not mean that there cannot be laws to restrict
smoking and the marketing of cigarettes, just as there are laws
against driving while intoxicated.

That is why the Surgeon General is such a hero. By taking a
stand with the health establishment, he speaks in a manner contrary
to the political philosophy of the powers to whom he is ultimately
responsible. The tobacco senators who oppose him will work un-
ceasingly, not so much to deny the truth in what he reports, for that
is really irrefutable. Rather they will seek to destroy his reputation
and then replace him with one of their own—a doctor who will
stop the flow of information to the public, saying that there are
problems more pressing than the question of people who die from
smoking cigarettes.

For the tobacco industry to enjoy continued success, it must
stop those reports.

The battle to control the sources of information is at the heart
of the struggle. The tobacco industry is seeking to cut off the flow
of information to the public; with the FTC, they succeeded in

stopping the annual reports after 1985. They know that the truth will ultimately destroy them. In preventing access to information on the tar/nicotine content of cigarettes, they make it more difficult for people to quit smoking. Their next step will be to get the testing stopped altogether.

The basic questions are very simple:

- Does the public have the "right to know" about less dangerous cigarettes?
- Does the government have an obligation to tell the public about less dangerous cigarettes?

Now that smoking has been shown to harm the nonsmoking public in the Surgeon General's report of 1985, the innocent by-stander has been shown to be the innocent victim. Smoking is now identified as a **public** health hazard, one that affects not just smokers, but everyone who breathes.

Specifically, the report states:

Chronic simple bronchitis has been associated with occupational exposure in both nonsmoking exposed workers and populations of exposed workers. ... Smoking has commonly been demonstrated to be the more important factor in producing these symptoms.[1] A pack of day smoker takes 50,000 puffs per year.[2]

THE NEXT STEPS

At the beginning of this book I said that the two things the cigarette industry fears most are an effective plan for quitting smoking, and government regulation.

I have tried to provide the first. In addition I have some ideas for people who want to act now.

1. Call Smokers What They Are: Addicts

It sound like a little thing, but smokers do not like to be called addicts: but that is what they are, addicts. Emphasize the fact

1. *Seventeenth Annual Surgeon General's Report; Cancer and Chronic Lung Disease in the Workplace, 1985, p. 13.*
2. *op cit., pg. 15–5.*

that they are addicts in all anti-smoking literature—that they are addicts, just like cocaine addicts. Emphasize this particularly in anti-smoking literature to children, so that they know that once they get started, it will be very difficult for them to stop.

2. Start at Home

Encourage your parents and other family members to quit smoking. If you are an adult, tactfully point out to your friends that their smoking is not healthy for their children and sets a bad example. Statistics show that a much higher proportion of children smoke if their parents smoke.

3. Pressure Employers at Work

Point out to your employer that if he does not take action to isolate smokers in special work areas, the Surgeon General's report lays him wide open to legal action. This is particularly true if his business involves any of the materials specifically covered in the 1985 Surgeon General's Report on smoking in the Workplace. The problem is two-fold: (a) The smoke from cigarettes gives co-workers bronchitis; and (b) Cigarette smoke in combination with many materials used in manufacturing can increase the odds that workers will get cancer.

The Surgeon General's report says flatly that programs to stop smoking at work are **more successful** than clinic-based programs. Higher cessation rates in worksite programs are achieved with more intensive programs. The report says that, "Incentives for nonsmoking appear to be associated with higher participation and better success rates." *

Some companies, such as U.S. Gypsum, have gone to the extent of forbidding employees to smoke **even at home** because of the greater health risks from the combination of cigarette smoke and the raw materials that workers must be in contact with at their jobs.

4. Let Businesses Know What You Want

(a) Restaurants, Stores and Airlines. There is nothing worse than a mouthful of smoke when you are trying to enjoy a dinner out or a

* Source: Surgeon General's Report of 1985; Cancer and Chronic Lung Disease in the Workplace.

drink at the bar on the way home. Urge restaurants to ban smoking, but if they will not, at least encourage them to have a separate smoking area. If they park a smoker next to you, complain and ask the management to give them a table far away from you. The airlines are obligated to give you a seat in a nonsmoking area, even if it means the smokers have to give up smoking. So, exercise your rights.

(b) *Shopping Malls, Theaters, Stores and Shopping Centers.* There is no reason anyone should have to inhale a lot of cigarette smoke every time they go into a local store or mall. Smoking in stores is not only a health hazard, it is a fire hazard as well. The same thing applies in enclosed shopping malls. Let smokers go outside and smoke. The other day I had a dress ruined at the Mid Island Mall by someone who was careless with a cigarette.

5. Raise Cigarette Taxes

Write your local newspaper and your politicians to raise the cigarette tax. This can be done at the state as well as the federal level.

The influence of the tobacco senators has caused the inflation-weighted price of cigarettes to drop. Today's price of $1.25 per pack is really only $.33 in 1968 dollars. The price of tobacco has gone up more than the price of cigarettes. Why are cigarettes relatively so much cheaper now than in the past? Because the tobacco industry is there with its contributions at election time, lobbying away against cigarette taxes, trying to keep the price down.

The record shows cigarettes increase our health costs. You and I pay that cost in our health insurance fees. We are paying for care for smokers' health problems caused by their addiction. If they don't want to give up cigarettes, tax them to pay the health bills.

Because the tobacco lobby has such a hold in Washington, the best place to put pressure is on your state legislature. Experience shows that even though some smokers quit, the extra money paid in taxes by those who continue more than makes up for the revenue loss to the states. So we should tax and tax, particularly now that we know the effects of smoking in the workplace and the damage it does to everybody's health.

After all, it is better than taxing gasoline, which is a necessity, or sports events, which are pure fun, or children's clothing, or medicines or a host of other things that contribute to our welfare and our pleasure. Smoking does nothing but hurt us. For years we have known that it injures their health; now we know that it injures our own.

Raise the cigarette tax. Make smokers pay the health costs.

6. Use Your Vote; Be Vocal

This is the most important step of all. No one wants to prohibit smoking, the sale of tobacco products or tobacco farming. That would be totally foolhardy. On the other hand, smoking injures both the smoker and the people nearby. Therefore there is ample justification for legal limits on its use around other people. Here are some of the places you can make your voice count.

(a) PTAs. The evidence is clear. No one is born with an urge to smoke. Children take it up because it symbolizes adulthood, macho behavior and because of peer pressure from their friends who have already become addicted.

Have your local PTA vote in favor of anti-smoking educational programs **starting in grammar school.** Local school districts are very sensitive to PTA pressures. Your local teachers know the dangers of smoking and do not want to see your children become addicted. The earlier you can turn your children away from cigarettes, the better.

(b) Town Halls. Get your city or town council to set an example. Smoking in the workplace injures the public and shouldn't be allowed. No one wants to restrict employees' rights, but let them smoke where they won't hurt other people.

(c) State and County Offices. Government issues the medical reports, and government should set the example. Smoking in public offices should be restricted or forbidden to keep down the cost of state and county employees' health insurance. Write or call your local repre-sentative, especially if you are a businessman. Politicians are par-ticularly responsive to business people because that is where their contributions come from.

7. Endorse Anti-Smoking Candidates

The most important thing any single person can do is to make his opinion felt around election time. Write a letter that states your position against smoking, and your interest in voting for legislators committed to that position; have five or ten or fifteen people sign it. Then send it in to the candidates who are running. This is the time when politicians are the most sensitive, because they need you and your vote. You will be surprised at how much attention your letter gets.

8. Endorse Restrictions on Cigarette Advertising

It is time that we faced the obvious. Cigarette smoking, not just a brand of cigarette, is sold through advertising. The symbolism used in the ads showing health adult, macho, peer group sports and status is what gets kids started on cigarettes in the first place. And once they start, they are hooked, many for life.

What particularly ticks me off both as a mother and as a marketing professional is the way they use clean, outdoor, healthy, young people's sports to promote their sales. It is not only the big, four-color magazine spreads, it is the promotion and the implied endorsements. The best example I can think of is that Virginia Slims tennis tournament. To use the clean, healthy kids that play tennis to promote cigarettes is outrageous, simply outrageous. And yet it is perfectly legal. And it is not just tennis, it is auto racing, jazz concerts, bike races, rock festivals and all the other activities that appeal to young people.

I know how well these promotions work, especially with children. I worked on the studies to test the effectiveness of their advertisements and promotional campaigns. The problem is that Congress just is not going to do anything to stop support of bike races, jazz concerts and tennis matches unless they hear from you, the voter, in a big way. So, do something: start writing and organizing.

Let us start with getting the promotions banned. It is going to be tougher getting the advertising banned because the media is so dependent on cigarette companies' spending.

Tobacco and smoking are completely legal and should remain so, but I feel there is no reason at all to make cigarettes **look** attractive. Why put such an addictive substance in an attractive package and give it a safe-sounding name?

Eventually, not immediately, but eventually, I feel cigarettes should be sold only in plain-wrap, generic-type packges. This would remove the ego identification from the brand names and greatly reduce the attractiveness of their use. There is nothing so subtle or vicious as the companies' use of image and ego appeals (which they do superlatively) to market their products.

I know. I used to test the effectiveness of their packages as well as their ads.

9. Force the Publication of Tar/Nicotine Data

This is, I think, the greatest sin. Here we have a known carcinogen, and the government has bowed to the pressure of the tobacco senators and refuses to release the information people need to know how to cut down on their habit.

I do not know how they get away with it. Yell, scream, write, call your congressman; do anything to get that data released so people will know how to cut down.

10. Support Measures to Put Cigarettes Under the FDA

This one is the toughest of all. The tobacco companies will fight it tooth and nail because it is potentially the single step that can cause them the most damage.

Like food and other drugs, tobacco is a substance people take into their bodies. The great advantage that the tobacco companies have other most other marketers of substances Americans take into their bodies is this: THEY ARE NOT UNDER THE FOOD AND DRUG ADMINISTRATION.

The Food and Drug Administration is the toughest, meanest agency in the government. They are intended to be that way because their whole purpose is to protect the health of the public. That is why you see a list of ingredients on the box of corn flakes. The tough stand of the FDA is why we never had the thalidomide babies. In Europe and Japan, where thalidomide was not regulated, birth defects were the unfortunate result; babies were born with flippers instead of arms. Even corn flakes have to pass inspection, because they are under the jurisdiction of the Food and Drug Administration.

But not cigarettes. Cigarettes are under the Bureau of Alcohol, Tobacco and Firearms, which is run by the Treasury Department. And the Treasury Department isn't interested in health; it is interested in money. The Treasury Department has a vested interest in the cigarette tax money.

Cigarettes are both a drug and a poison. They should be put under the jurisdiction of the Food and Drug Administration.

Conclusion

The giant tobacco companies have enormous resources with which to do battle, but in the long run a politician has to get elected and to do that he needs your support. That is why we ask you to write and to act. If you do not, the tobacco companies will slowly throttle the sources of public information, and the people will continue to get hurt.

It is no accident that the highest proportion of smokers are less-well-educated, blue-collar Blacks (about 50 percent usage) and whites, while the better-educated professional, technical and kindred workers have the lowest rates of current smoking (approximately 26 percent), according to the 1985 Surgeon General's report.

The tobacco companies prey on the poor and the less well educated, taking money from their pockets every day of their lives. After all, if we were all brilliant and perfectly disciplined, there would be no need to organize and ask the government's help in restricting smoking. But we do not live in a perfect world, and a cigarette is a dreadful temptation.

I know, because I too was once humilated by my own inability to give them up—and sometimes I have trouble resisting temptation even now.